About the Authors

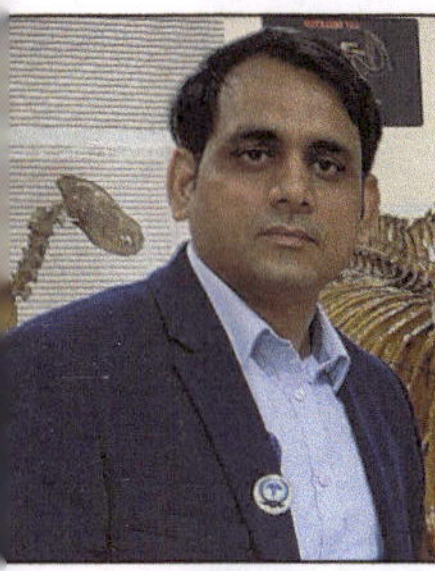

Dr. Abhinov Verma is Assistant Professor in Department of Veterinary Anatomy, College of Veterinary Science and Animal Husbandry, DUVASU, Mathura (UP) and has engaged in undergraduate and postgraduate teaching from the last 10 years. He Published 52 research papers in various national and international journals, 62 abstracts, 07 popular articles, 08 manuals and 06 book chapters. He received IAVA Young Scientist Award, Best Paper and Poster Presentation awards in various conferences; Best PhD Thesis Award by DUVASU, Mathura, Teaching Excellence Award by AEDS, Best Veterinarian Award by The Science World Magazine and Dr. B.V.Rao Poultry Entrepreneurs Global Icon Award by Pashudhan Praharee. He is Reviewer of various national & international journals. He is Editorial Board Member of Indian Journal of Veterinary Anatomy, HSOA Journal of Animal research and Veterinary Science, The Science World and Journal of Veterinary Reviews. He is Registered Veterinary Practitioner of UPVC affiliated with VCI. He is Life member of various scientific societies like Indian Association of Veterinary Anatomists (IAVA), Electron Microscope Society of India, ISSGAPU and Society for Immunology and Immunopathology. He attended more than 30 national and international symposium/conferences/webinars and 16 national/international trainings. He has handled various intramural as well as extramural projects.

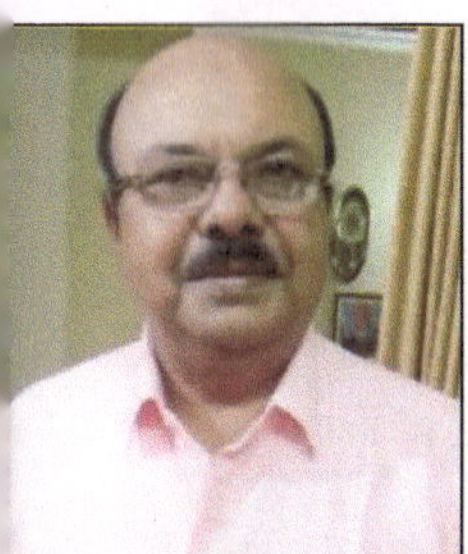

Dr. Ajay Prakash is Professor in Department of Veterinary Anatomy, College of Veterinary Science and Animal Husbandry, DUVASU, Mathura and has engaged in undergraduate and postgraduate teaching from the last 32 years. He published more than 120 research papers in various national and international journals, 160 abstracts, 18 popular articles, 16 manuals and 04 book chapters. He received Fellow of Indian Association of Veterinary Anatomists, IAVA Anatomist of the year award, many Best Paper and Poster presentation awards in various conferences. He is Life member of various scientific societies like Indian Association of Veterinary Anatomists (IAVA), Indian Association of Animal Production and Indian science congress. He attended more than 32 national and international symposium/conferences. He guided 05 M.V.Sc, 02 Ph.D students and act as member of advisory committee of 16 students. . He was Secretary, Member of editorial board, Member of executive committee of Indian Association of Veterinary Anatomists. He chaired various administrative posts like Head of the department, President Games and sports, Estate Officer, Chief Personnel Officer, Establishment officer, Director Farms and Dean Post graduate studies in DUVASU,Mathura.

Bovine Myology
A Colour Atlas

NIPA® GENX ELECTRONIC RESOURCES & SOLUTIONS P. LTD
New Delhi-110 034

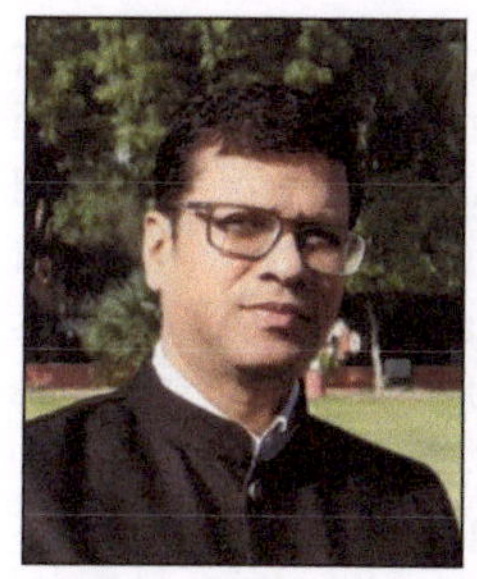

Dr. Shriprakash Singh is Associate Professor in Department of Veterinary Anatomy, College of Veterinary Science and Animal Husbandry, DUVASU, Mathura and has engaged in undergraduate and postgraduate teaching from the last 14 years. He had published 67 research papers, one book, 11 manuals, 2 review articles, 27 semitechnical articles, 10 folders and 7 chapters' in different books. He developed a mobile app on the Veterinary Histology. He guided 2 PG students as Chairman; and member of advisory committee in 6 PG and PhD students. He organized National seminar in 2011, winter school sponsored by ICAR in 2018 as member of core committee and 2023 as coordinator. He acts as organizing secretary in User Awareness sessions on National Digital Library of India. He received NAVS (I) membership award in 2021. He also received many Best Paper and Poster Awards in various conferences. He received National level awards for the Hindi scientific article and Dr. B.V.Rao Poultry Entrepreneurs Global Icon Award by Pashudhan Praharee. Dr. Singh has very successfully carried out the administrative responsibilities in the university as Hostel warden, Establishment officer, Public information officer Recruitment Officer.

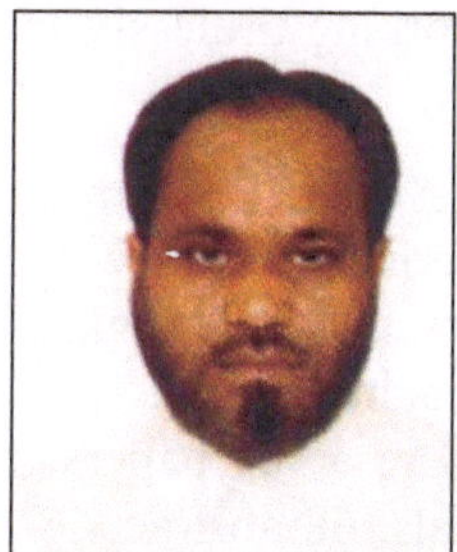

Dr. MM Farooqui is Professor in the Department of Veterinary Anatomy, College of Veterinary Science and Animal Husbandry, DUVASU, Mathura and has engaged in undergraduate and postgraduate teaching from the last 33 years. He published more than 120 research papers in various national and international journals, 160 abstracts, 15 popular article, 16 manuals and 06 book chapters. He received Fellow of Indian Association of Veterinary Anatomists, Award for Best paper published in Indian Journal of Veterinary Anatomy, Many best papers and poster presentation awards in various conferences, Award for best PhD thesis guided (02) and Best Teacher Award by DUVASU, Mathura. He is Life member of Indian Association of Veterinary Anatomists (IAVA). He attended more than 20 national and international symposium/conferences. He guided 03 M.V.Sc, 03 Ph.D students and act as member of advisory committee of more than 15 students. He chaired various administrative posts like Head of the Department, Dean Student Welfare and Establishment officer in DUVASU, Mathura.

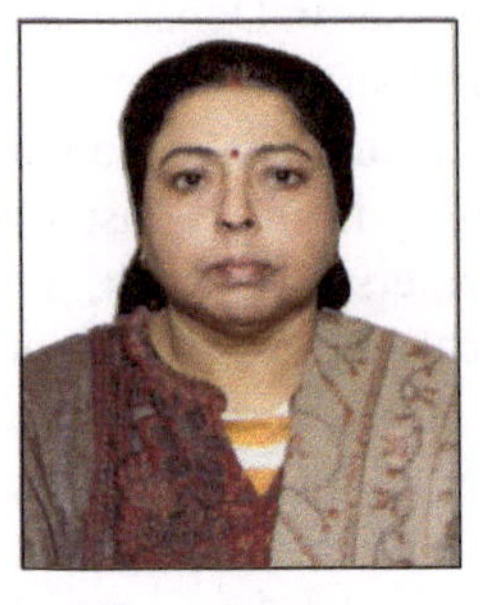

Dr. Archana Pathak is Professor and Head, Department of Veterinary Anatomy, College of Veterinary Science and Animal Husbandry, DUVASU, Mathura and has engaged in undergraduate and postgraduate teaching from the last 25 years. She has guided two M.V.Sc. and two Ph.D theses as Major Advisor and a number of post-graduate students as a co-guide. She has published 130 research articles in the journals of national and international repute, 08 book chapters, 20 teaching/training manuals and 8 semi-technical articles. She is a distinguished Fellow of National Academy of Veterinary Science, India (NAVS-I), Fellow of Indian Association of Veterinary Anatomists (IAVA) and has been honoured with several national awards such as Young Scientist Award and Gold Medal of Indian Association of Veterinary Anatomists; Award of Indian Association for the Advancement of Veterinary Research (IAAVR) for the recognition in research contributions in Veterinary Anatomy; Member of NAVS-India; Dr. P.S. Lalitha Silver Jubilee Award & Medal for the Best Paper published in Indian Journal of Veterinary Anatomy and several other Best Paper awards. She is life member of several scientific societies. Her research works have been recognized at national and international levels. She is still working tirelessly for the promotion of teaching and research in Veterinary Anatomy.

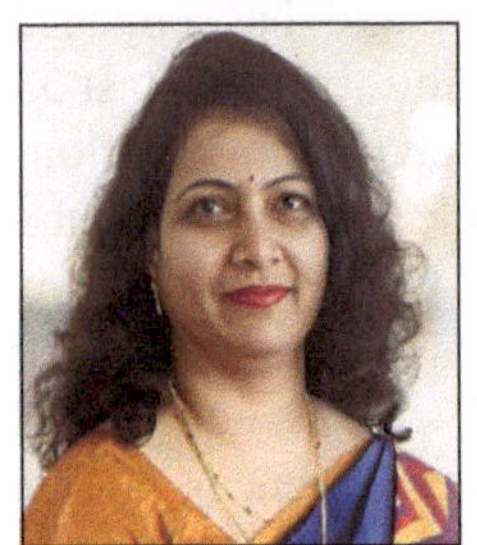

Dr. Varsha Gupta is Associate Professor in the Department of Veterinary Anatomy, College of Veterinary Science and Animal Husbandry, DUVASU, Mathura and has engaged in undergraduate and postgraduate teaching since from the last 14 years. She has Published 60 research papers in various national and international journals, 68 abstracts, 02 popular articles, 02 review articles, 11 manuals, and 06 book chapters. She has received IAVA Best PhD Thesis Award, Best Paper, and Poster Presentation awards in various national and international conferences, best M.V.Sc. Thesis guided award. She had guided one M.V.Sc student and was a member of 05 M. V. Sc. Students. She has participated in 12 National and International trainings, 4 International and 20 National conferences. She is a member of different veterinary societies like the Indian Association of Veterinary Anatomists, the Indian Poultry Science Association, Indian Society for sheep and goat production and utilization, etc. The author has also organized the national conference of IAVA, 21 days of Winter school by ICAR, webinars, and quizzes in various capacities.

Bovine Myology
A Colour Atlas

Abhinov Verma
Assistant Professor
Department of Veterinary Anatomy
College of Veterinary Sciences and Animal Husbandry
DUVASU, Mathura, Uttar Pradesh

Ajay Prakash
Professor
Department of Veterinary Anatomy
College of Veterinary Sciences and Animal Husbandry
DUVASU, Mathura, Uttar Pradesh

Shriprakash Singh
Associate Professor
Department of Veterinary Anatomy
College of Veterinary Science and Animal Husbandry
DUVASU, Mathura, Uttar Pradesh

M. M. Farooqui
Professor
Department of Veterinary Anatomy
College of Veterinary Sciences and Animal Husbandry
DUVASU, Mathura, Uttar Pradesh

Archana Pathak
Professor and Head
Department of Veterinary Anatomy
College of Veterinary Sciences and Animal Husbandry
DUVASU, Mathura, Uttar Pradesh

Varsha Gupta
Associate Professor
Department of Veterinary Anatomy
College of Veterinary Sciences and Animal Husbandry
DUVASU, Mathura, Uttar Pradesh

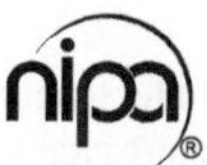

NIPA® GENX ELECTRONIC RESOURCES & SOLUTIONS P. LTD.
New Delhi-110 034

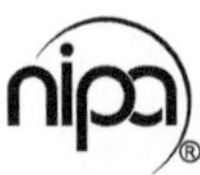

NIPA® GENX ELECTRONIC RESOURCES & SOLUTIONS P. LTD.

101,103, Vikas Surya Plaza, CU Block
L.S.C.Market, Pitam Pura, New Delhi-110 034
Ph. +91 11 27341616, 27341717, 27341718
E-mail: newindiapublishingagency@gmail.com
www: www.nipabooks.com

For customer assistance, please contact
Phone: + 91-11-27 34 17 17
Fax: + 91-11-27 34 16 16
E-Mail: feedbacks@nipabooks.com

ISBN: 978-93-58876-49-9

Composed and Designed by NIPA®.

Preface

In the view of its importance in surgical, physiological and clinical fields this book has been prepared to provide basic knowledge of Veterinary Myology for the Undergraduate and Post Graduate Students. The aim of this colour atlas was to compile a work of this kind for the guidance of the students in dissection skills. This colour atlas is as per the guidelines of Veterinary Council of India. Although books on Veterinary Myology of different species of animals are accessible but no colour atlas with illustrations on Bovine Myology is available. The efforts have been made to publish a full illustrated dissection guide to understand the intricate lacing of different muscles in their original natural position. The book contains information on muscles of different regions of the body with their origin, insertion, action, blood and nerve supply. The authors acknowledge Dr. Prabhakar Kumar, Professor, SVPUAT, Meerut for their valuable suggestions, Mr. Akhil Gupta (2nd Professional B.V.Sc. & A.H. student) for sketch diagrams.

Authors

Contents

List of Colour Plates

List of Tables

1

Introduction of Myology

Myology: It is the branch of biological science which deals with the description of different muscles and their accessory structures.

Muscle is a contractile tissue present in all animals. Its function is to produce motion. Impulses from nerve cells control the contraction of each muscle fiber. Contractile part of muscles is muscular tissue.

There are three kinds of muscular tissue in the body:

a. Striated or striped muscle

b. Non-striated or unstriped or smooth muscle

c. Cardiac muscle.

For dissection purpose only striated muscles are included in this book.

Striated Muscles

Striated muscles are for most part connected directly or indirectly with the skeleton, upon which they act, and are hence, designated as skeletal or somatic muscles.

Skeletal muscles cover the greater part of the skeleton, and thus in a large measure determine the form of animal. They are red in color, the shade varying in different muscles and under various conditions. Red colour of a muscle is due to the presence of myoglobin. When myoglobin is more in the muscles, they are designated as red muscles. When myoglobin is less in the muscles, they are classified as white muscles. Some skeletal muscles are intimately associated with the skin are called cutaneous muscles. Muscular part of each is composed of bundles of contractile fibers surrounded by a thin sheath of connective tissue- the perimysium.

Description of Skeletal Muscle

It is convenient to divide the description of a muscle into following seven heads-

(1) Name (2) Shape and Position (3) Attachments (4) Action (5) Structure (6) Relations (7) Blood and Nerve Supply

1. The Name

It is determined by the various considerations, i.e. action, attachment, shape, position and the direction etc. In most cases two or more of these factors are combined to produce the name, e. g., Flexor carpi radialis, longus colli and obliquus abdominis externus.

2. The Shape and Position

Shape is, in many cases, sufficiently definite to allow the use of such terms as triangular, quadrilateral, fan-shaped, fusiform and ring-like, etc. Some muscles vary greatly in form, and may be classified as long; broad, short and flat etc. Orbicular or ring-like muscles circumscribe orifices which they close, hence are termed sphincters. Position is usually stated with reference to the region occupied and to adjacent structures which may be presumed to be already known.

3. The Attachments

The attachments are in most cases to bone, but many muscles are attached to cartilage, ligaments, fascia, the skin, etc. Usually the term origin is applied to the attachment which always or more commonly remains fixed when the muscle contracts. The term insertion designates the more movable attachment. With respect to the muscles of the limbs the proximal attachment is regarded as origin and the distal one as the insertion. In all cases the attachment is by means of fibrous tissue, the muscle-fibers not coming into direct relation with the point of attachment. But when intermediate fibrous tissue is not evident to the naked eye, i.e. perimysium of muscle is fused directly with periosteum or perichondrium, it is customary to speak as a fleshy attachment. Term tendinous attachment is applied to those cases in which intermediate fibrous tissue, tendons or aponeurosis, is evident. Tendon is a band of dense white fibrous tissue by means of which a muscle is attached. An aponeurosis is a broad fibrous sheet which fulfils a similar requirement.

4. The Action

The action of muscle belongs chiefly to physiological study. Muscle which concur in action are termed synergists, those which has opposite actions are antagonists. Following terms are generally used in regard with the action-

1. Flexion- Action in which angle between the bones / parts is decreased.
2. Extension- Action in which angle between the bones / parts is increased.
3. Adduction - When two limbs come close to each other.
4. Abduction - When two limbs go away from each other.

5. The Structure

It includes direction of the muscle-fibers, arrangement of tendons, the synovial membranes, and any other accessory structures, e.g., annular ligaments and reinforcing sheaths and bands. The terms fleshy and tendinous are used to indicate the relative amounts of muscular and fibrous tissue. When muscle is fusiform, the large fleshy part is often spoken of as the belly (Venter) of the muscle.

In the case of the long muscles of limbs, the origin is often termed the head. Muscles having two or more heads are named biceps, triceps, etc. Digastric muscles are those which have two bellies joined by an intermediate tendon. Ring-like muscles which circumscribe openings are termed sphincters, on account of their action.

Muscles may have parallel arrangement of fibres (Fig. 1.1). Muscles may have spindle shaped or fusiform shape arrangement in which fibers converge upon a tendon at both ends of muscle. In most of the cases the muscle fibers join the tendon at an acute angle, hence, term pennate is used to indicate this arrangement. A muscle in which the fibers converge to either side of the tendon is termed bipennate. Muscle in which this arrangement exists only on one side of the tendon is called unipennate. More complex arrangement is resulting in a multipennate muscle. Some muscles are intersected by tendinous layers or bands known as tendinous intersections. The intersecting bands or tracts which appear on the surface usually as Zig-zag lines are termed tendinous inscriptions.

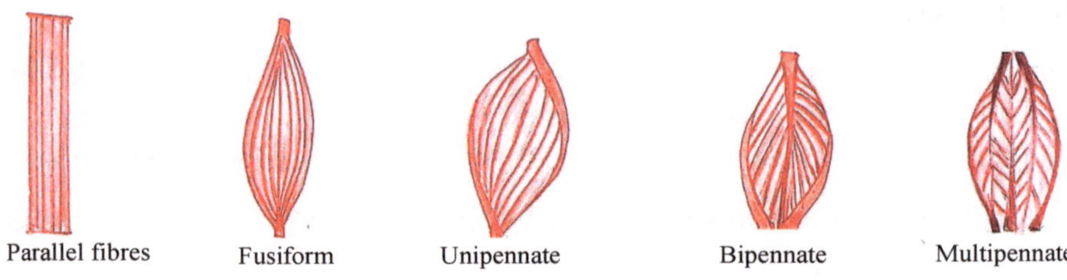

Fig. 1.1: Diagrams of Various Arrangements of Skeletal Muscles Fibers

6. Relations

The relations of muscle constitute an important part of topography and are very important on surgical ground.

7. Blood and Nerve-Supply

These are of clinical interest. The muscles have a large blood supply. The nerves to the muscles are motor, sensory, and vasomotor in function.

The Accessory Structures

The accessory structures are as follows

1. Synovial membranes
2. Fasciae

1. Synovial Membranes

The synovial membranes are arranged in two principal forms: (a) Synovial bursa (b) Synovial sheath.

Synovial bursa (Bursa mucosa) is a simple sac interposed at a point of unusual pressure between tendon or muscle and some deeper seated structure, most commonly a bony prominence. Bursa occur in certain situations between the fascia and underlying structures (subfascial bursa), or between the fascia and the skin (subcutaneous bursa). Synovial sheath or Tendon sheath differs from a bursa in the fact that the synovial sac is folded around the tendon more or less completely, so that two layers can be distinguished. Inner layer adheres closely to the tendon, while the outer lines the groove or canal in which the tendon lies. Two layers are continuous along a fold termed the mesotendon.

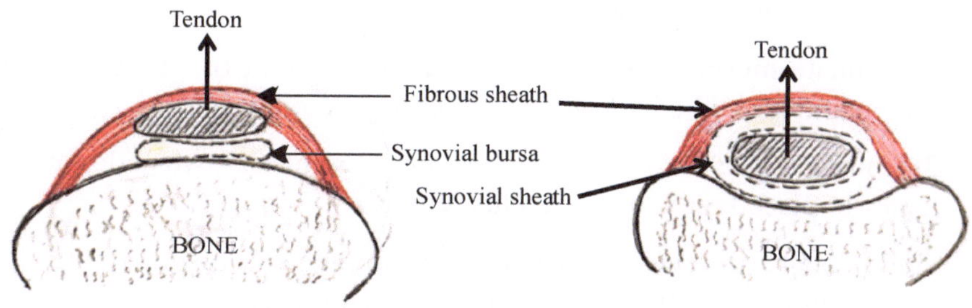

Fig. 1.2: Diagrams of Cross Section of Synovial Bursa (A), Synovial Sheath (B)

2. Fasciae

These are sheets of connective tissue, mainly of the white fibrous variety, with a greater or less admixture of elastic fibers in certain cases.

Usually two layers of faciae are present

1. Superficial fascia (Fascia subcutanea) is composed of loose connective tissue which may contain more or less fat and is subcutaneous.
2. Deep fascia composed of one or more layers of dense fibrous tissue spread over the surface of the muscles chiefly.

Many muscles are enclosed in fibrous sheaths which hold them in position.

Classification of Muscles

Muscles can be classified as follows

I- According to the Colour of Muscle

A) **Red muscles-** Having relatively more amount of myoglobin.

B) **White muscles-** Having relatively less amount of myoglobin. They are less red and are generally superficial.

II-According to the arrangement of muscle fibers

A) **Parallel muscles**- Fibers are less in number but are long and are placed parallel to the line of pull. eg. Biceps brachii

B) **Fusiform muscles -** Fibers converge upon a tendon at both ends of the muscle.

C) **Pennate muscles-** Fibers joins the tendon at an acute angle like the barbs of a feather to its central axis.

i) Unipennate muscles- All muscle fibers are present on one side of the tendon and look like half of the feather. eg. Peroneus tertius.

ii) Bipennate muscles- Muscle fibers are present on two sides of the centrally placed tendon. eg. Rectus femoris

iii) Multipennate muscles- More complex arrangement in which fibers join the tendon from multiple directions. eg. Deltoideus

D) **Spiral muscles-** Fibers are arranged in a twisted manner. eg. Brachialis

E) **Cruciate Muscles-** Fibers are arranged in superficial and deep planes crossing like X. eg. Masseter

III- According to the Force of Action

A) **Spurt muscles-** Produce acceleration movement to the joint. eg. Brachialis

B) **Shunt muscles-** Produce stabilizing centripetal force on a joint. eg. Flexor carpi radialis

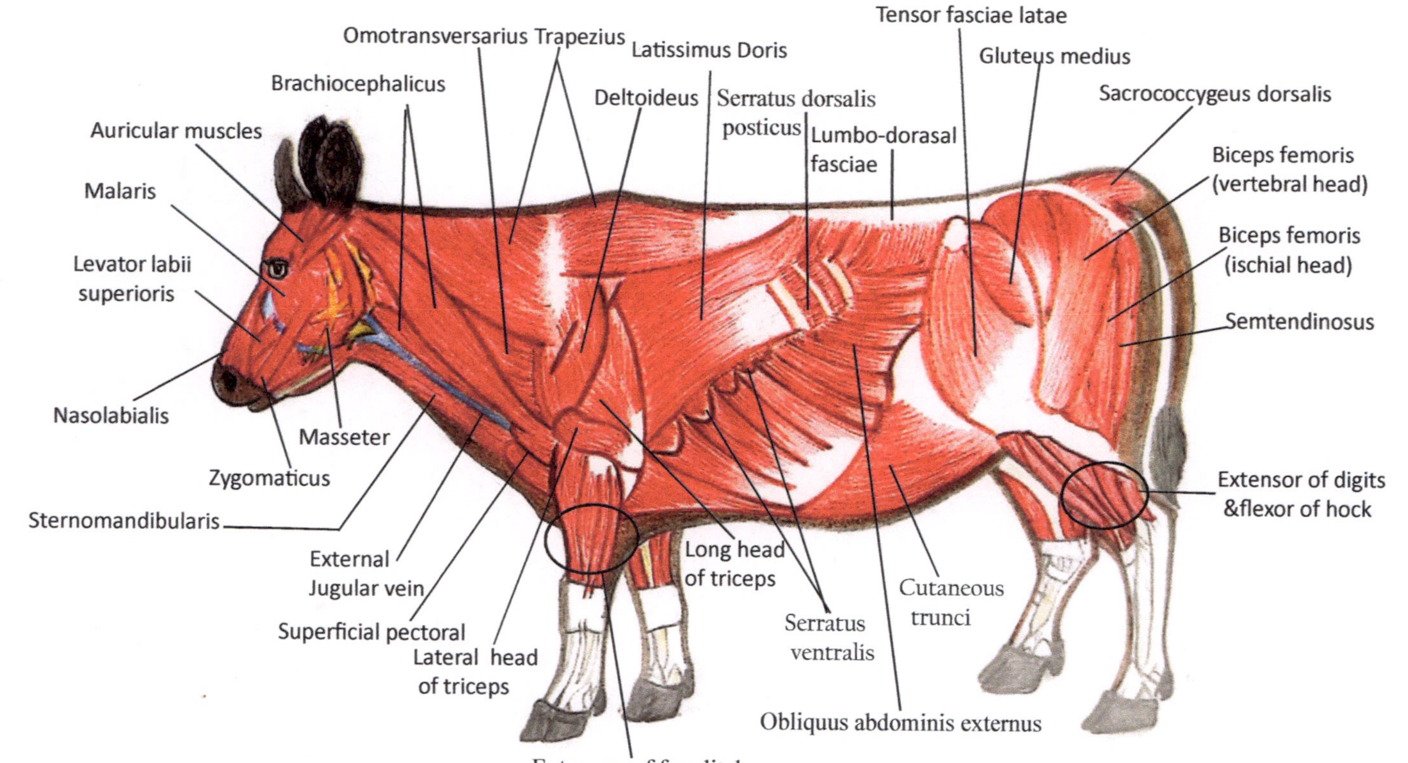

Fig. 1.3: Diagram of Superficial Musculature of Bovine

2

Muscles of Shoulder and Arm Region (Lateral Aspect)

Site of incision: Make a straight dorso-ventral incision through skin from the summit of dorsal vertebral spine to the cranioventral aspect of shoulder joint. Extend it up to the cranial margin of shoulder joint, then caudo-ventrally up to caudal most part of elbow joint. Make another ventrodorsal straight incision from caudal most point of elbow joint to the summit of vertebral spine then reflect the skin flap from ventral to dorsal up to mid dorsal line of the body. Remove the facia to expose the various muscles of this region.

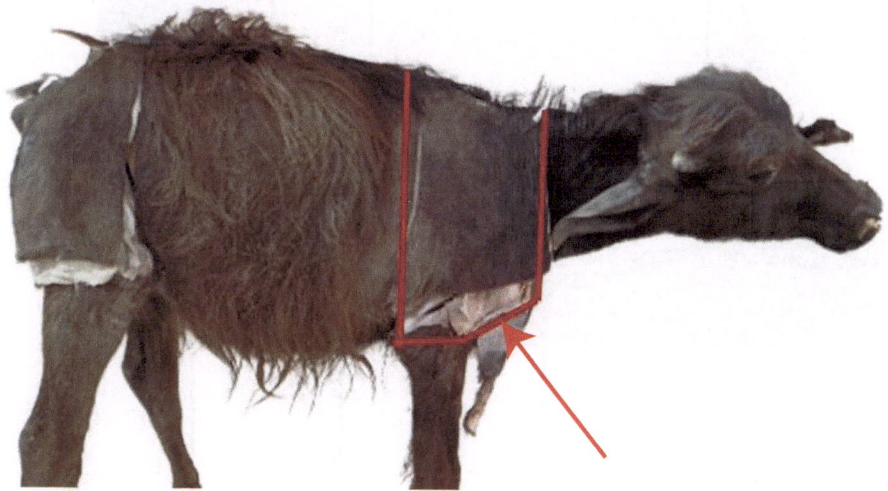

Fig. 2.1: Site of Incision for muscles of shoulder and arm region (lateral aspect)

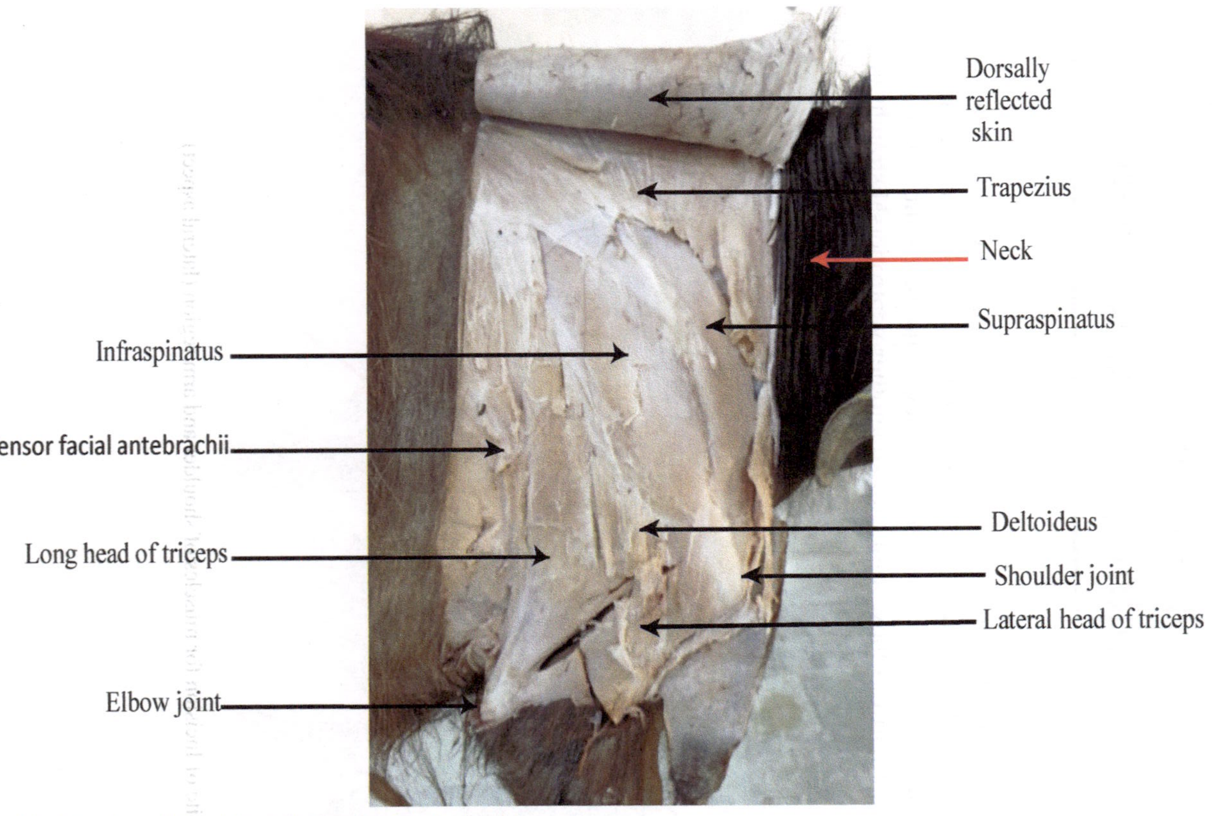

Fig. 2.2: Muscles of Shoulder and Arm Region (Lateral Aspect)

Table 2.1: Detail of Muscles of Shoulder and Arm Region (Lateral Aspect)

S.N.	Name of Muscle	Origin	Insertion	Action	Blood and Nerve supply
1.	Supraspinatus*[1]	Suprapinous fossa, cartilage of scapula and spine of scapula	Anterior parts of the medial and lateral tuberosities of the humerus.	Extend the shoulder joint	Suprascapular and posterior cervical arteries Suprascapular nerve.
2.	Infraspinatus	Infraspinous fossa, scapular cartilage and spine of the scapula	Medial surface of posterior part of the lateral tuberosity and a circular rough area below the anterior part of the lateral tuberosity of the humerus.	Abduct the arm and possibly to rotate it outward and also serves as the lateral collateral ligament of the shoulder	Subscapular artery Suprascapular nerve
3.	Deltoideus*[2]	Acromion process and adjacent part of the scapular spine, the scapular spine by the aponeurosis covering the infraspinatus muscle and the upper part of the posterior border of the scapula.	Deltoid tuberosity and the brachial fascia of the arm	Flex the shoulder joint and abduct the arm	Posterior circumflex artery of the humerus and subscapular artery Axillary nerve
4.	Teres minor*[3]	Distal half of the posterior border of the scapula	The deltoid tuberosity and small area just above it	Flex the shoulder joint	Posterior circumflex artery of the humerus and the subscapular artery. Axillary nerve

S.N.	Name of Muscle	Origin	Insertion	Action	Blood and Nerve supply
5.	Long head of triceps	Posterior border of the scapula	Lateral and posterior part of summit of olecranon	Flexes the shoulder joint and extend artery of the elbow joint	Subscapular, triceps branch of the posteri- or circumflex artery of the humerus and of th humerus and deep brachial arteries. Radial nerve
6.	Tensor facia ante-brachii	Tendon of insertion of latissimus dorsi	Deep fascia and the olecra-non.	Flex the shoulder and extend the elbow joints	Subscapular and thoraco-dorsal artery Radial nerve
7.	Lateral head of triceps	A curved muscular line above the deltoid tuber-osity	Lateral surface of olecranon and the antibrachial fascia.	Extend the elbow	Similar to long head of triceps
8.	Brachialis[*4]	Proximal third of posterior surface of humerus	Medial border of radius	Flex the elbow joint	Posterior circumflex artery of the humerus. Musculocutaneous branch of the median nerve.

*1. Dorsal part of this muscle is covered by the trapezius whereas the ventral half is covered by brachiocephalicus and omotransversarious (both muscles discuss with muscles of neck region).

*2. This muscle has two parts: acromion part and scapular part and in between the two parts the infraspinatus muscle is present.

*3. To expose this muscle scapular part of deltoideus is cut as it is located below this part.

*4. This muscle is present in musculospiral groove of humerus under the lateral head of triceps brachii muscle.

3

Muscles of Pectoral Region

Site of incision

Remove the skin flap of pectoral region to expose the pectoral muscles.

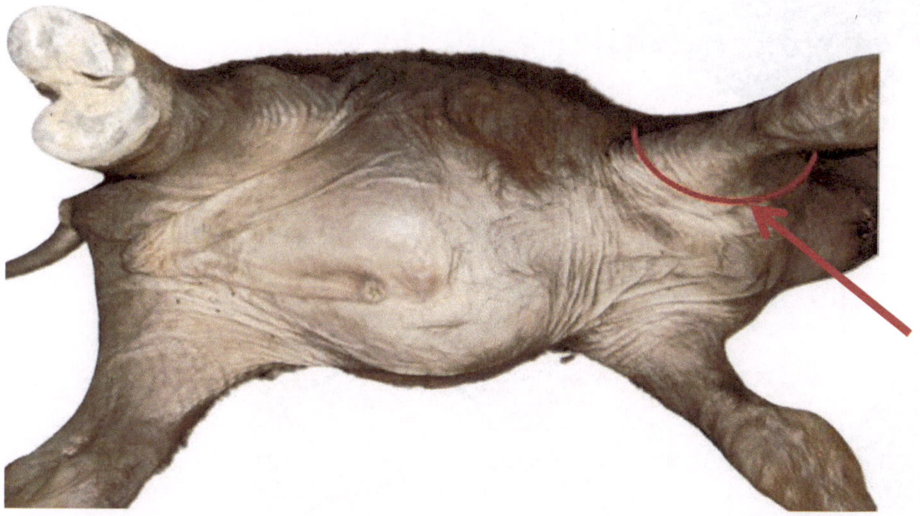

Fig. 3.1 Site of Incision for Muscles of Pectoral Region

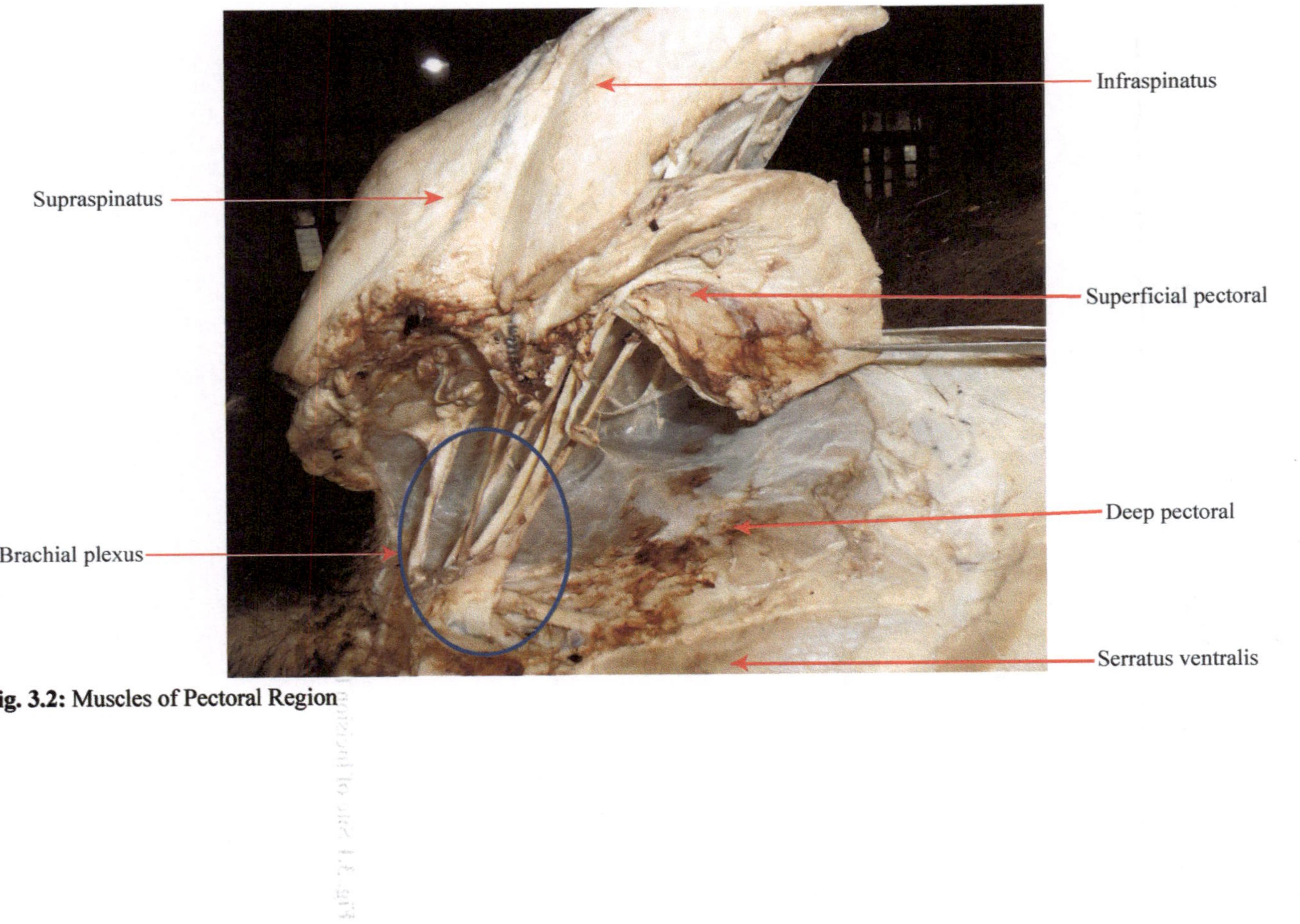

Fig. 3.2: Muscles of Pectoral Region

Table 3.1: Detail of Muscles of Pectoral Region

SN	Name of muscle	Origin	Insertion	Action	Blood and Nerve supply
1.	Superficial pectoral	Anterior surface of the manubrium and ventral surface of the sternum to the level of the fourth sternebra and a median raphe common to the right and left muscles.	Distal part of the humeral crest below the insertion of the brachiocephalicus and the fascia on the medial surface of the forearm	Chiefly adduction of the limb. When the limb is advanced, to pull the body forward or to retract the limb.	External thoracic artery Pectoral nerves
2.	Deep pectoral/ Pectoralis profundus	Ventral surface of the sternum, a median raphe and the abdominal tunic.	Medial surface of the medial tuberosity and the anterior margin of the lateral tuberosity of the humerus.	To draw the trunk forward in walking or to retract the limb.	External thoracic artery. Pectoral and external thoracic nerves.

Note: After cutting the muscles of pectoral region we can access the brachial plexus

4

Muscles of Shoulder and Arm Region (Medial Aspect)

Site of incision: Detach the limb from the trunk by cutting various muscles viz; pectoral muscles, serratus ventralis, latissimus dorsi, brachiocephalicus, omotransversarius, trapezius, rhomboideus and long head of triceps.

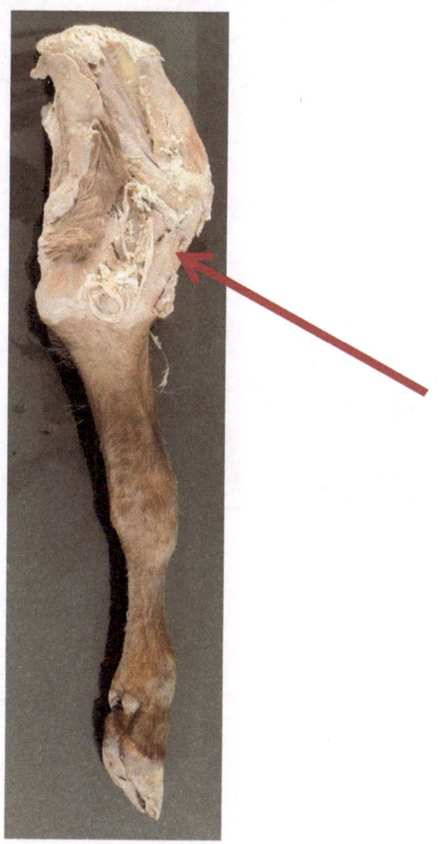

Fig. 4.1: Site of exposer for Muscles of Shoulder and Arm Region (medial aspect)

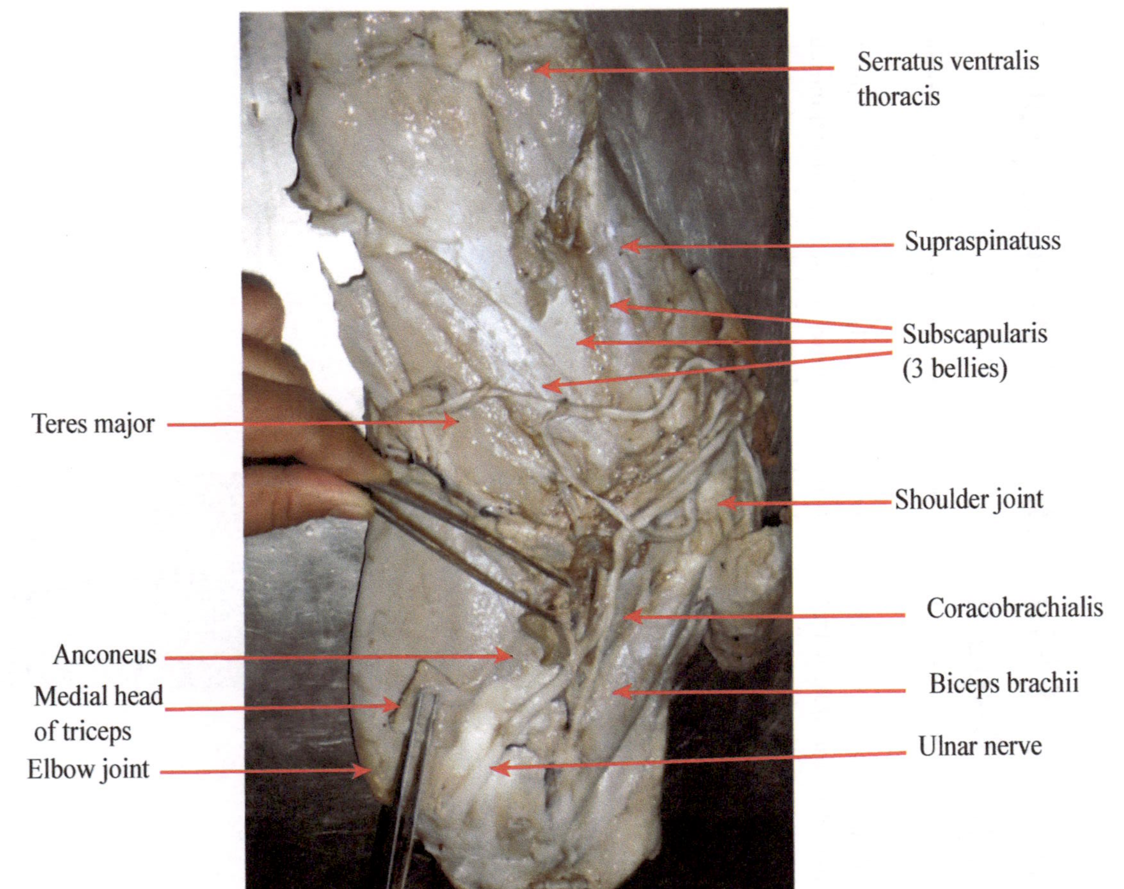

Fig. 4.2: Muscles of Shoulder and Arm Region (Medial aspect)

Table 4.1: Detail of Muscles of Shoulder and Arm region (Medial Aspect)

S.N	Name of muscle	Origin	Insertion	Action	Blood and Nerve supply
1.	Subscapularis	Costal surface of the scapula and scapular cartilage	Posterior part of medial tuberosity of the humerus	Adduct the limb.	Subscapular artery and circumflex artery of the scapula Subscapular and axillary nerves
2.	Teres major	Posterior angle and a little of the adjacent posterior border of the scapula	Teres tuberosity of the humerus with the latissimus dorsi muscle	Flex the shoulder joint	Subscapular artery Axillary nerve
3.	Coracorbrachialis	Coracoid process of scapula	1. Small area above the teres tubercle of humerus 2. Middle third of anterior surface of humerus	Adduct the arm and flex the shoulder joint	Anterior circumflex artery of humerus Musculocutaneous nerve
4.	Biceps brachii	Tuber scapulae	Radial tuberosity, medial ligament of the elbow joint, tendon of the pronator teres and the antibrachial fascia	Flex the elbow joint, extend and fix the shoulder joint, assist in extending the carpus and tense the dorsal antibrachial fascia	Anterior circumflex artery of humerus and a muscular (bicipital) branch from brachial artery Musculocutaneous nerve
5.	Triceps brachii (medial head)	Medial surface of the humerus just below the head	Posterior surface of the olecranon and the antibrachial fascia	Extend the elbow	Subscapular, triceps branch of the posterior circumflex artery of humerus and deep brachial artery Radial nerve

6.	Anconeus	Posterior surface of the humerus and the ridges forming the boundaries of the olecranon fossa	The anterior border and lateral surface of the olecranon.	To extend the elbow joint. The posterior part of the joint capsule is attached to this, thus raised above the articular surface which prevents it from being pinched when the joint is extended	Subscapular artery Radial nerve
7.	Serratus ventralis thoracis	Lateral surfaces of first eight or nine ribs	Caudal triangular area on costal surface of scapula and adjacent part of cartilage	Raise the thorax	Deep cervical, vertebral and dorsal intercostal arteries V to VIII cervical nerves and long thoracic nerve

Note: In Addition to above muscles the Muscle Supraspinatus is also visible from the Medial Aspect cranial to the Subscapularis Muscle.

5

Muscles of Extensor Group of Fore Limb

Site of incision

Make a mid-lateral and mid-medial longitudinal incision on forelimb from elbow joint to 3rd digit. Joins the above incisions transversally on cranial aspect of elbow joint and 3rd phalanx, respectively. Remove the skin on dorsolateral aspect of limb

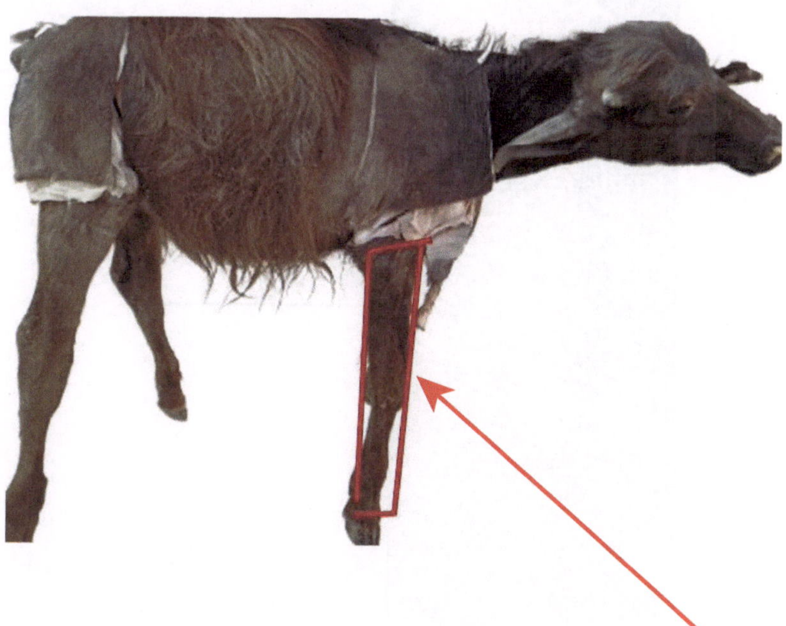

Fig. 5.1: Site of Incision for Muscles of Extensor Group of Fore Limb

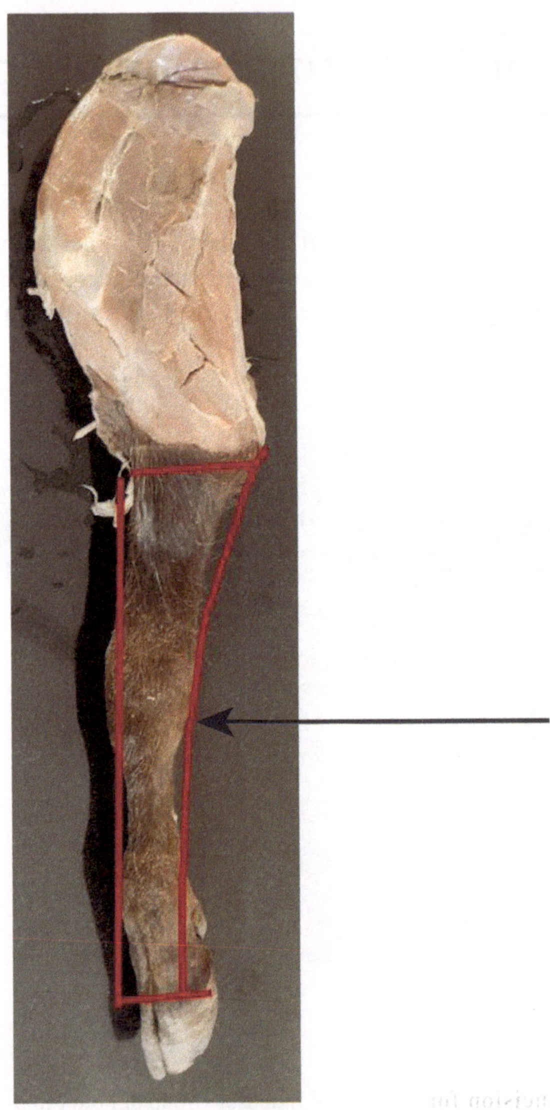

Fig. 5.2: Site of Incision for Muscles of Extensor Group of Fore Limb

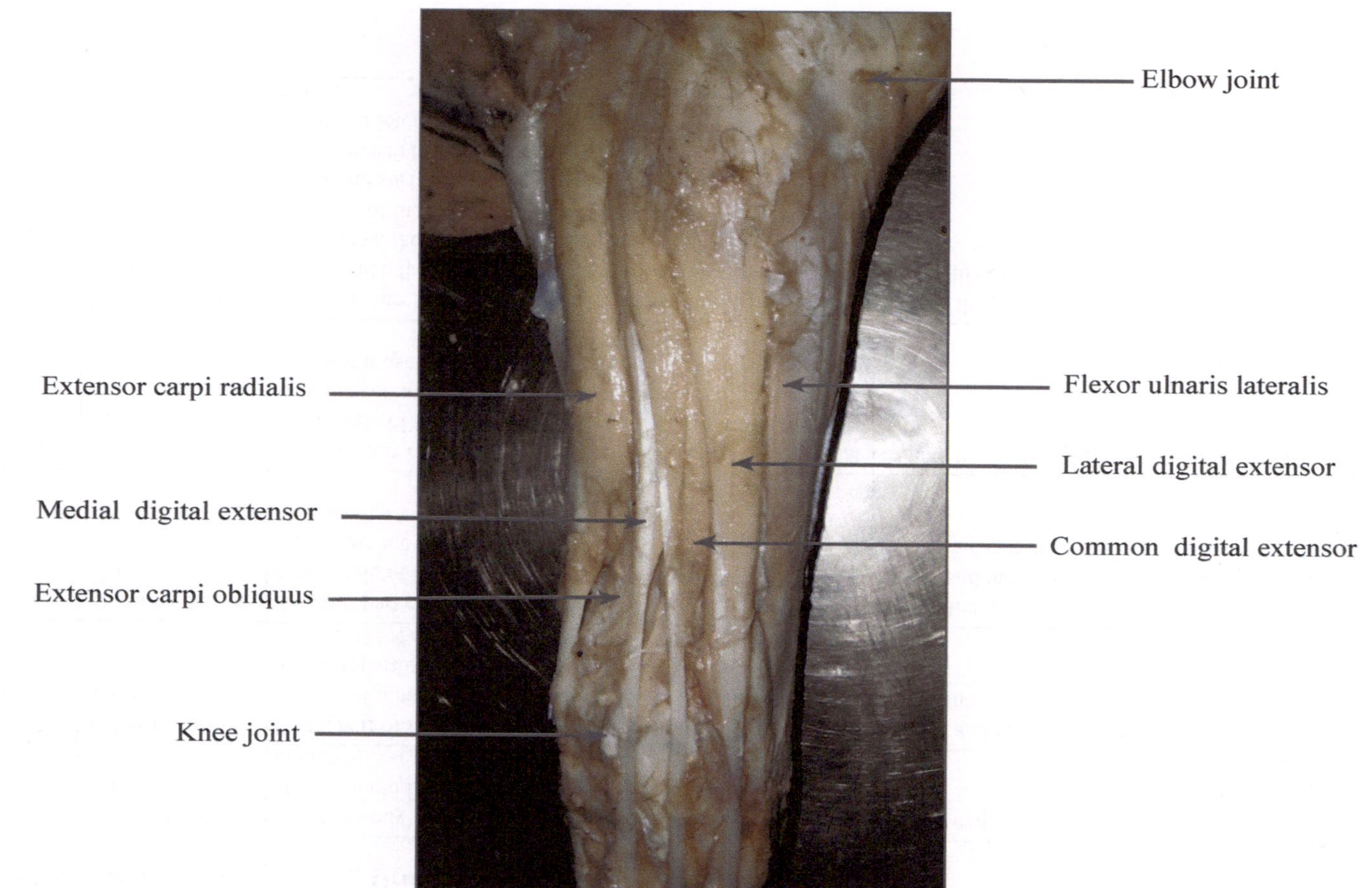

Fig. 5.3: Muscles of Extensor Group of Fore Limb

Table 5.1: Detail of Muscles of Extensor Group of Fore Limb

S.No.	Name of muscle	Origin	Insertion	Action	Blood and Nerve supply
1.	Extensor carpi radialis	Lateral condyloid crest and coronoid fossa of the humerus	Metacarpal tuberosity	Extend carpus and flex the elbow	Radial artery and radial nerve
2.	Extensor carpi obliquus	Distal half of lateral surface of ulna and adjacent part of the dorsal surface of the radius	Mediovolar angle of proximal extremity of large metacarpal	Extend and possibly slightly rotate outward the carpal joint	Dorsal interosseous artery and nerve
3.	Common digital extensor	Anterior part of lateral epicondyle of humerus and lateral surface of shaft of ulna above the interosseous space	Extensor process of third phalanx of both digits	Extent the digits, flex the elbow and indirectly to extend the carpus.	Radial artery Radial nerve
4.	Medial digital extensor	Anterior part of the lateral epicondyle of the humerus with the common digital extensor muscle	Anterior border of the proximal extremity of the second phalanx and abaxial part of the articular border of the third phalanx of the third digit.	Extend the pastern joint and abduct the digit	Radial artery and radial nerve
5.	Lateral digital extensor	Lateral tuberosity of the radius and adjacent part of the ulna, the lateral ligament of the elbow and the lateral surface of the ulna between the proximal and distal interosseous spaces.	Anterior part of the proximal extremity of the second phalanx and the abaxial part of the articular border of the third phalanx of the lateral digit.	Extend the pastern joint and abduct the digit	Common interosseous artery and radial nerve

6

Muscles of Flexor Group of Fore Limb

Site of incision- Make a mid-lateral and mid-medial longitudinal incision on forelimb from elbow joint to 3rd digit. Join the above incisions transversally on caudal aspect at elbow joint above and 3rd phalanx below, respectively. Remove the skin on palmero-medial aspect of limb.

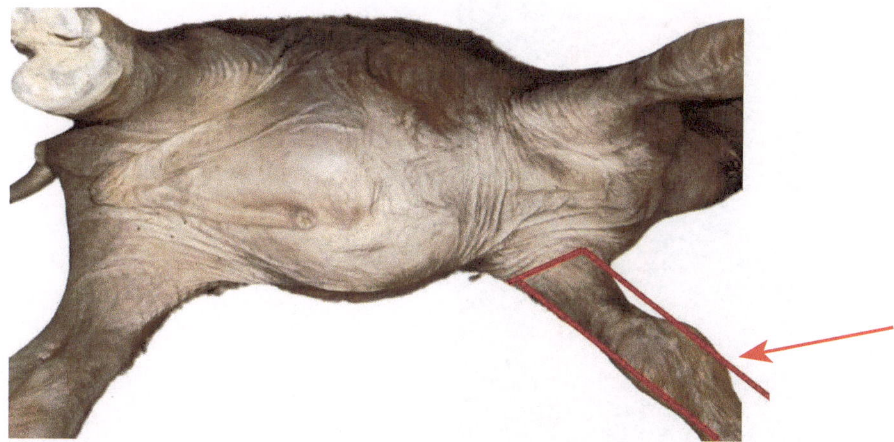

Fig. 6.1: Site of incision for Muscles of Flexor Group of Fore Limb

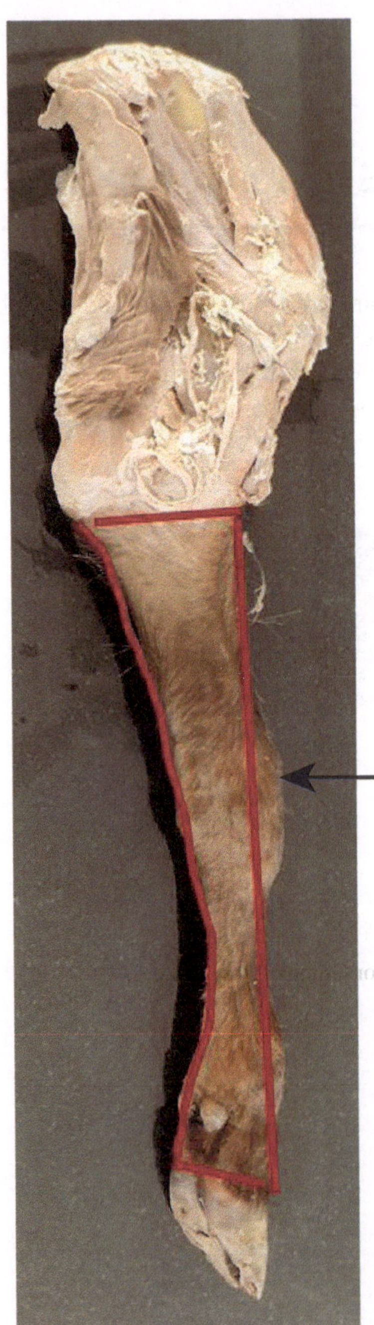

Fig. 6.2: Muscles of Flexor Group of Fore Limb

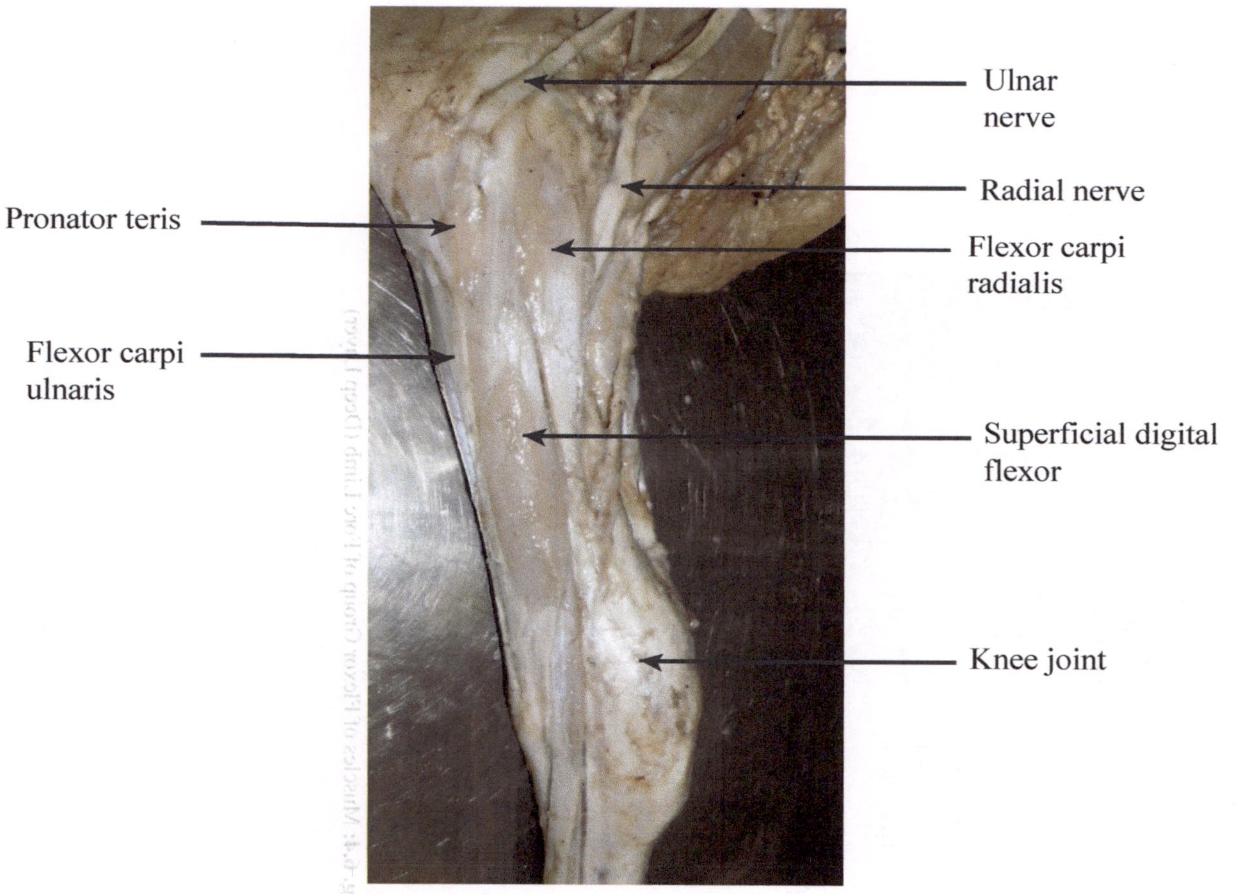

Fig. 6.3: Muscles of Flexor Group of Fore Limb (Superficial Layer)

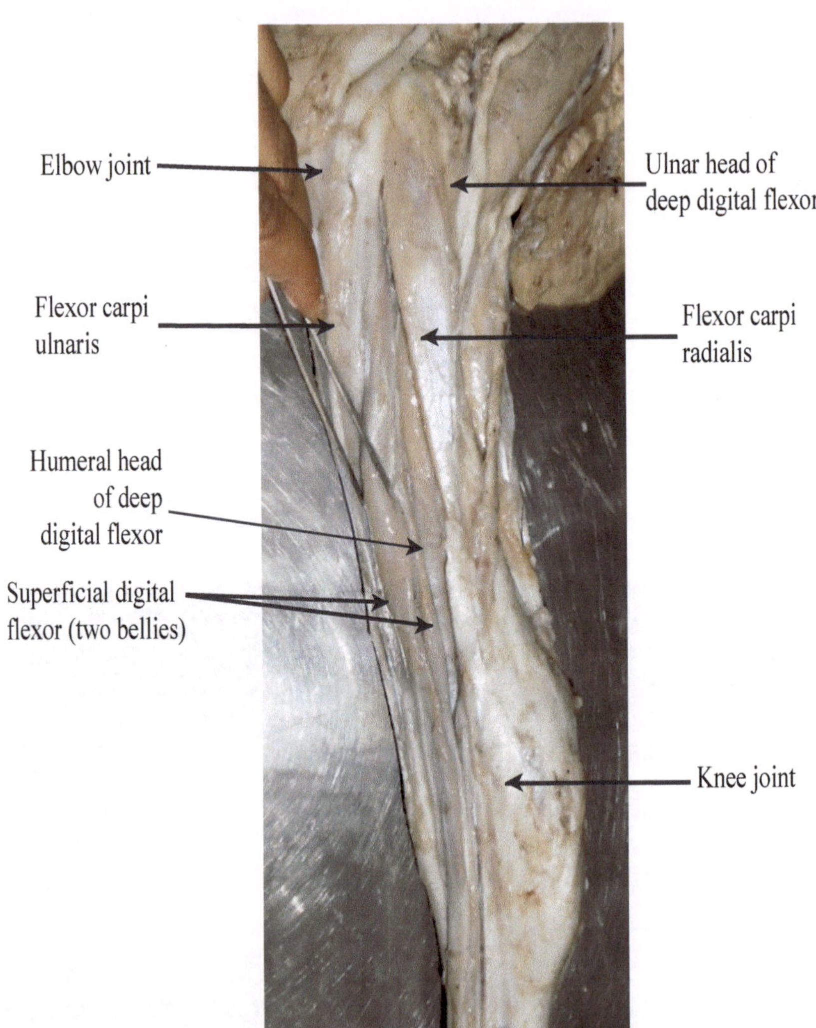

Fig. 6.4: Muscles of Flexor Group of Fore Limb (Deep Layer)

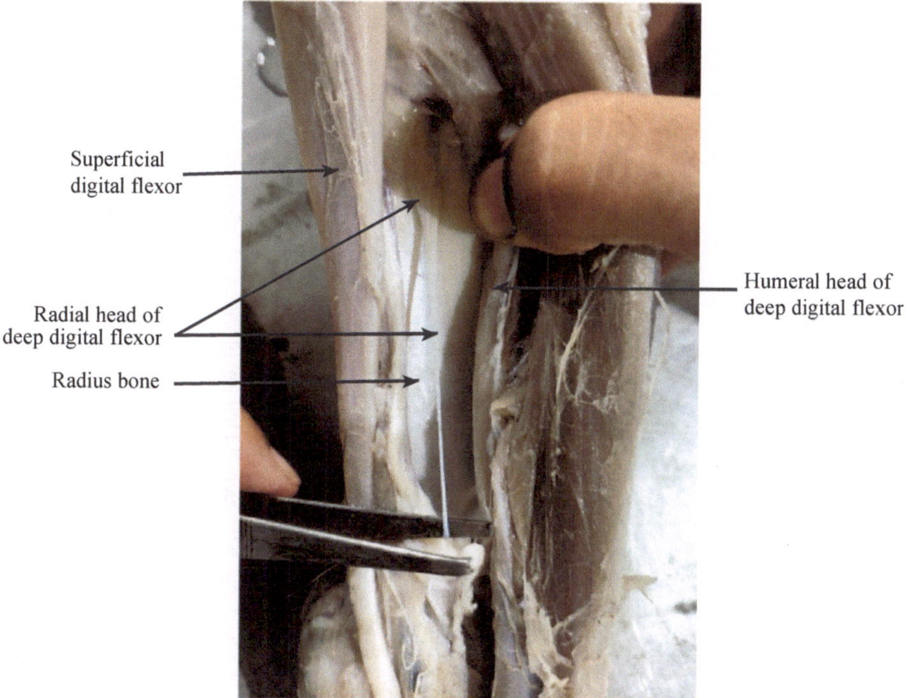

Fig. 6.5: Muscles of Flexor Group of Fore Limb (Deep Layer)

Table 6.1: Detail of Muscles of Flexor Group of Fore Limb

S.No.	Name of muscle	Origin	Insertion	Action	Blood and Nerve supply
1.	Pronator teres	Medial epicondyle of the humerus with the medial ligament of the elbow joint	Medial border of the radius	Probably no motion is produced	Median artery and median nerve
2.	Flexor carpi radialis	Medial epicondyle of the humerus just posterior to the medial ligament of the elbow	Postero-medial angle of the proximal extremity of the large metacarpal	Flex the carpal joint	Median artery and median nerve
3.	Flexor carpi ulnaris	Medial epicondyle of the humerus behind the origin of the flexor carpi radialis muscle and the medial surface of the olecranon	Posterior surface of the accessory carpal bone	Flex the carpus and slightly extend the elbow	Median and ulnar arteries and ulnar nerve
4.	Flexor ulnaris lateralis	Lateral epicondyle of the humerus	Lateral surface of the accessory carpal bone and a tubercle on the dorso lateral surface of the large metacarpal	Flex the carpal joint. It also has a slight extension action on the elbow joint	Interosseous artery and radial nerve
5.	Superficial digital flexor (02 fleshy belly	Medial epicondyle of the humerus	Volar border of the proximal extremity of the second phalanx of each digit	Chief action is to flex the digit on the metacarpus. Lesser actions are to flex the carpus and extend the elbow	Median artery Ulnar and median nerves
6.	Deep digital flexor (03 heads i.e. humeral, ulnar and radial head)	Medial epicondyle of the humerus, the medial and lateral surfaces of the ulna below the olecranon and the palmer surface of the radius on the level of the proximal interosseous space.	Palmer border of the third phalanx of each digit.	Flex the coffin joint, flex the digit on the metacarpus, to slightly extend the elbow and indirectly, to flex the carpal joint.	Median artery Ulnar and median nerves

7

Muscles of Lateral Aspect of Face Region, Lip and Cheek

Site of incision-Make a rostro-caudal incision along the ventral border of horizontal ramus of mandible then extend cranio-dorsally along caudal margin of nostrils up to middorsal line of face. From the caudal end of 1st incision make another incision dorsally up to base of the ear then passes cranially along the ventral aspect of eye up to mid dorsal line of face. Reflect the skin carefully from ventral to dorsal, carefully remove the muscle zygomaticus, malaris and nasolabialis as these are firmly attached to skin.

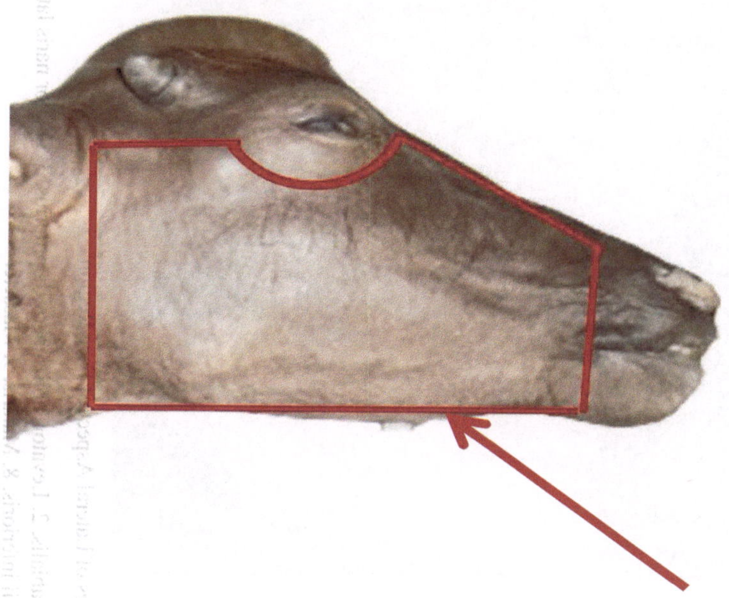

Fig. 7.1: Site of Incision for Muscles of Lateral Aspect of Face Region

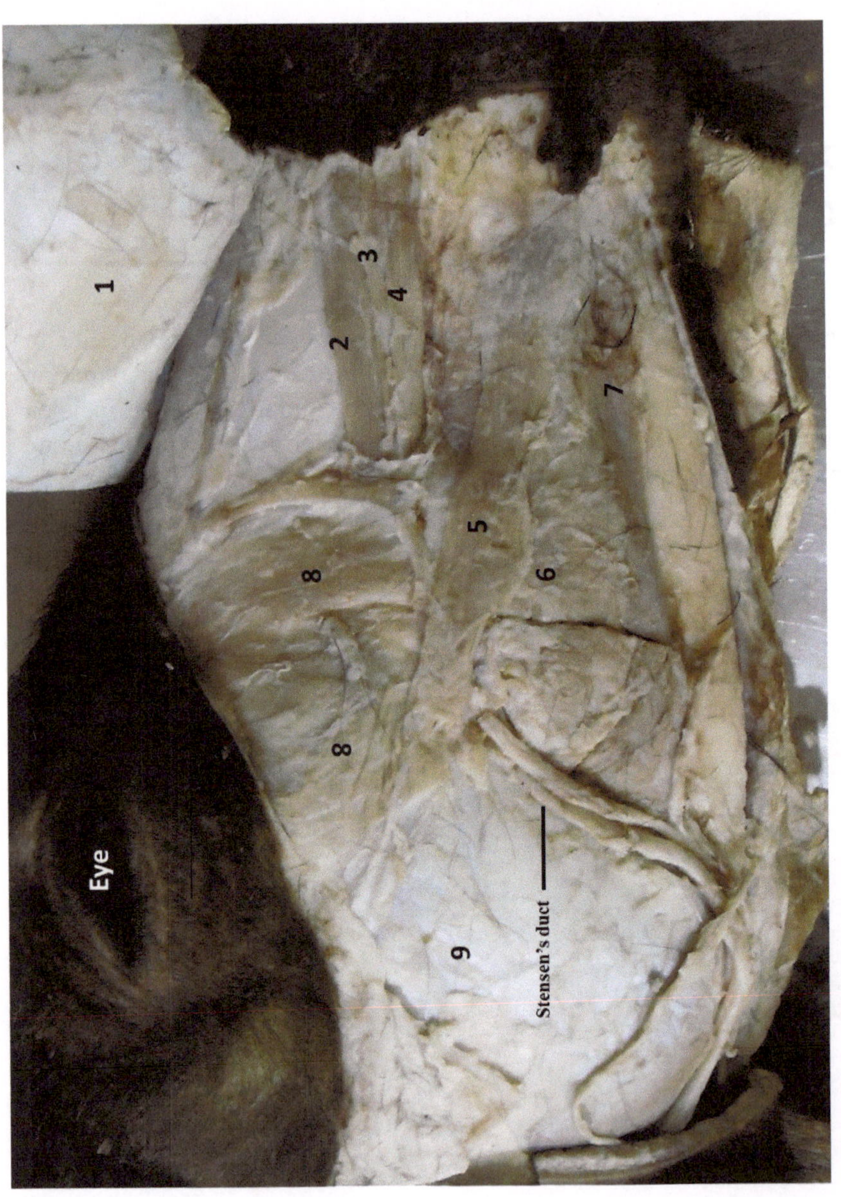

Fig. 7.2: Muscles of Lateral Aspect of Face Region

1. Levator nasolabialis, 2. Levator labii superioris proprius, 3. Dilator naris lateralis, 4. Depressor labii superioris, 5. Zygomaticus, 6. Buccinator, 7. Depressor labii inferioris, 8. Malaris, 9. Masseter

Table 7.1: Muscles of Lateral Aspect of Face Region, Lip and Cheek

S.N	Name of muscle	Origin	Insertion	Action	Blood and Nerve supply
1.	Levator nasolabialis	Nasal and anterior part of the frontal bone and the frontalis muscle.	Zuperficial layer inserts into the upper lip and the lateral part of the nostril. The deep part has an indefinite attachment to the lateral part of the nostril.	Slightly raise the upper lip and the lateral part of the nostril	Facial, dorsal labial and malar artery Facial nerve
2.	Levator labii superioris proprius	Facial tuberosity	To the central part of the upper lip by a flat tendon common to the right and left muscles	Slightly elevate the muzzle and with it the upper lip	Dorsal labial artery and facial nerve
3.	Zygomaticus	Zygomatic process of the malar bone, ventral to the lateral canthus of the eyelids	Angle of the lips where it blends with the orbicularis oris	Retract the angle of the lips	Facial artery and Facial nerve
4.	Dilator naris lateralis/Caninus	Facial tuberosity	Lateral wall of the nostril	To pull the lateral walls of the nostril outward the backward	Dorsal labial artery and Facial nerve
5.	Depressor labii Superioris	Anterior surface of the facial tuberosity	Anterior surface part of the upper lip and ventral part of the nostril	Retract the anterior part of the upper lip and adjacent part of the nostril	Dorsal labial artery and Facial nerve
6.	Depressor labii inferioris	Alveolar border of the mandible behind the last cheek tooth.	Lower lip and skin of the chin	Depress and retract the lower lip and chin	Superficial ventral labial artery and Facial nerve
7.	Buccinator	Alveolar borders of the maxilla and mandible from the level of the angle of the lips to where the alveolar border of the mandible turns upward.	Angle of the lips. Many of the superficial fibres pass from the upper to the lower jaw and have no definite insertion	Flatten the cheek thus pressing the food between the teeth and also to retract the angle of the mouth.	Deep ventral, dorsal labial and buccinators arteries Facial nerve

S.N	Name of muscle	Origin	Insertion	Action	Blood and Nerve supply
8.	Malaris a. Anterior malaris (Levator buccalis)	Facial part of the lacrimal bone.	Buccal mucosa ventral to the facial tuberosity	Raise the posterior part of the cheek..	Malar artery and Facial nerve
	b. Posterior malaris (Depressor palpebra inferioria)	Deep masseteric fascia over the anterior part of the masseter muscle.	Lower eyelid blending with the orbicularis oculi.	Depress the lower eyelid to open and widen the palpebral fissure.	Malar artery and Facial nerve
9	Masseter	Zygomatic arch and Facial crest	Lateral surface of the vertical part of the ramus of the mandible	Close the jaw and to move the mandible forward. When One muscle acting alone produces some lateral motion	External maxillary, transverse facial, masseteric, deep temporal arteries and Masseteric nerve
10.	Orbicularis oris	Sphincter muscle of mouth consists of two parts labial and marginal. Labial part continuous with other muscles which converge to the lips. Marginal part runs parallel to free edges of lips.		To close the lips	Facial, mental and palatolabial artery Facial nerve

8

Muscles of Mandible Tongue and Hyoid

Site of incision

Remove the skin of intermandibular space.Then remove one of the rami of mandible by disarticulating temporo-mandibular joint at caudal end and cut the ramus just behind the mental foramen.

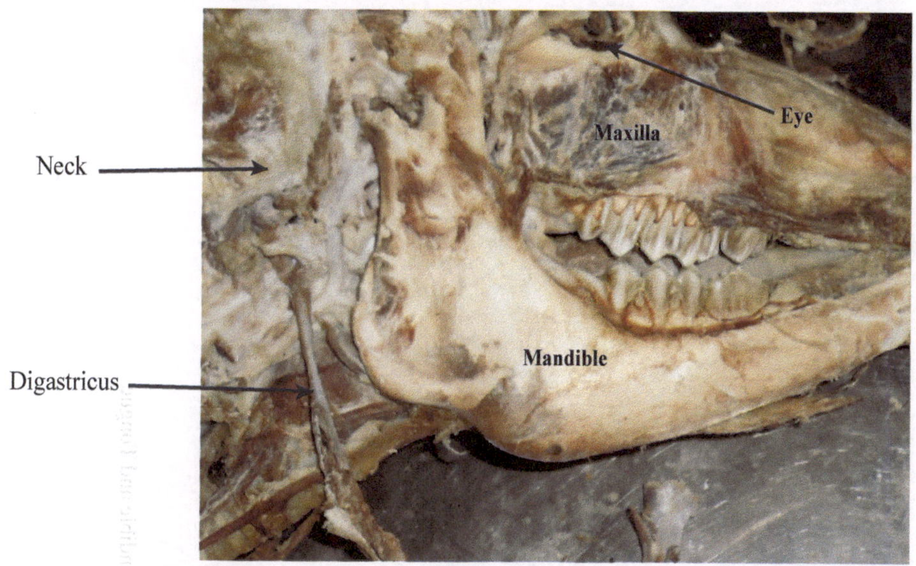

Fig. 8.1: Muscles of Mandible

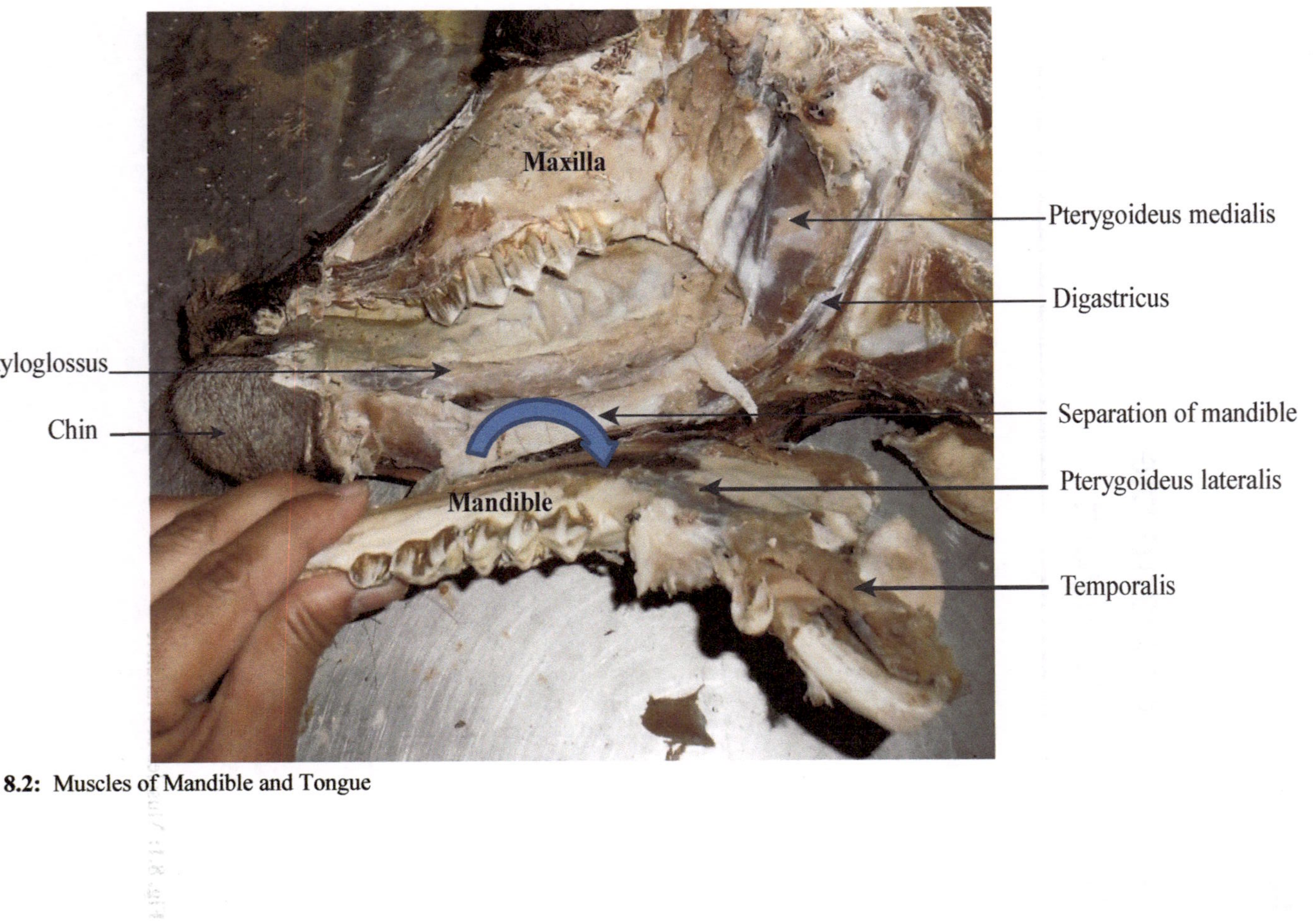

Fig. 8.2: Muscles of Mandible and Tongue

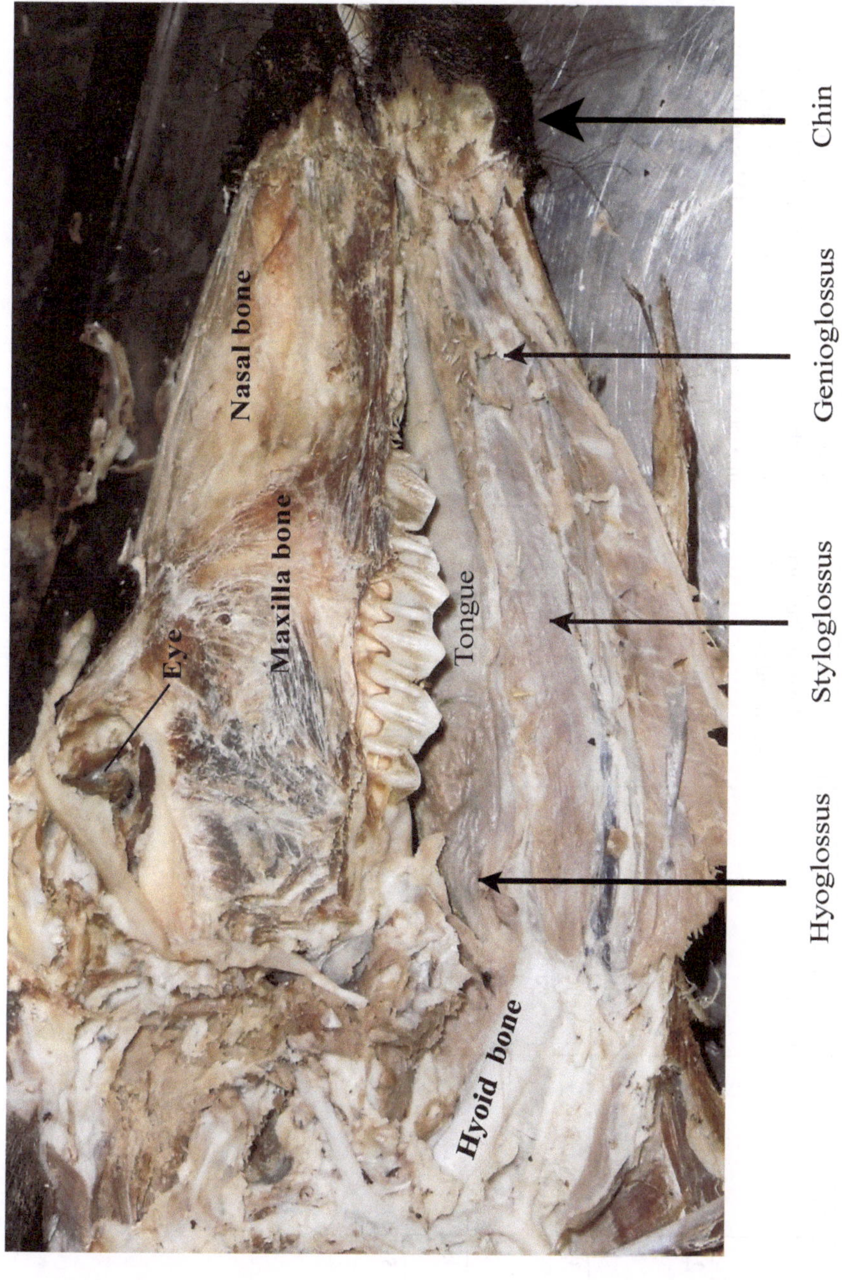

Fig. 8.3: Muscles of Tongue

Table 8.1: Detail of Muscles of Mandible

S.N	Name of muscle	Origin	Insertion	Action	Blood and Nerve supply
1.	Masseter	Zygomatic arch and Facial crest	Lateral surface of the vertical part of the ramus of the mandible	Close the jaw and to move the mandible forward. When One muscle acting alone produces some lateral motion	External maxillary, transverse facial, masseteric, deep temporal arteries and Masseteric nerve
2.	Pterygoideus medialis	Pterygoid process of sphenoid bone and lateral surface of perpendicular part of palatine bone	Medial surface of the mandible below and behind the mandibular foramen	Raise the lower jaw and also produce lateral movement of jaw	One or two pterygoid arteries from the internal maxillary. Pterygoid branches of the mandibular nerve
3.	Pterygoideus lateralis	Lateral surface of the pterygoid process of the sphenoid bone	Medial part of the anterior border of the mandibular condyle and adjacent part of the neck of the mandible	Move the mandible forward and also produce lateral motion to opposite side	Pterygoid artery and nerve
4.	Temporalis	Temporal fossa and temporal crest	Coronoid process and adjacent border	Raise the lower jaw	Deep temporal artery Mandibular nerve
5.	Digastricus	Paramastoid process of occipital bone	Medial surface of the horizontal ramus of the mandible close to the ventral border.	Depress the lower jaw and thus open the mouth. Possibly to retract the mandible after it has been protruded by the lateral pterygoid muscle.	External maxillary artery Mylohyoid and facial nerves

Table 8.2: Detail of Muscle of Tongue

1.	Styloglossus	Lateral surface of the great cornua of hyoid bone near the articulation with small cornua	Tip of the tongue	Retract and shorten the tongue	Lingual and sublingual branches of external maxillary artery Hypoglossal nerve, lingual nerve and glosso-pharyngeal nerve
2.	Hyoglossus	Lateral aspect of hyoid bone, from lingual process of great cornu and from thyroid cornu	Dorsum of the tongue	Retract and depress the tongue	
3.	Genioglossus	Angle of chin from medial surface of mandible just caudal to symphysis	To Intrinsic musculature	The muscle as a whole is depressor of the tongue	

Table 8.3: Detail of Muscles of hyoid

1.	Mylohyoideus	Medial surface of the mandible just below the alveolar border and the interdental space	Lingual process of the hyoid bone and median fibrous raphae	To raise the tongue, hyoid bone and floor of the mouth	Sublingual artery, Mylohyoid nerve
2.	Geniohyoidus	Posteroventral part of the symphysis mandibulae with the genioglossus muscle	Body of the hyoid bone	Draw the hyoid bone forward and protrude the tongue	Lingual and sublingual arteries, Hypoglossal nerve
3.	Stylohyoideus	The muscular angle of the hyoid bone	Lateral extremity of the body of the hyoid bone.	Draw the body of the hyoid bone back-ward and upward.	External maxillary artery Facial nerve
4.	Occipitohyoideus	Lateral surface of the paramastoid process	The puosterior border of the muscular angle of the hyoid bone	Draw the muscular angle backward and depress the anterior part of the hyoid bone.	Posterior auricular artery Facial nerve
5.	Keratohyoideus	The posterior border of the small cornu	The dorsal border of the thyroid cornu	To raise the thyroid cornu and with it the larynx	Lingual artery Lingual branch of the glossopharyngeal nerve

6.	Cervicohyoideus* (Omohyoideus)	Transverse process of the third and fourth cervical vertebrae.	Extremity of the body of the hyoid bone.	To raise/retract the hyoid bone.	Thyrolaryngeal artery and second cervical nerve.
7.	Sternothyrohyoideus*	Anterior surface of the manubrium sterni	Hyoid part, sternohyoideus, inserts on the body of the hyoid bone. The thyroid part, sternothyroideus, attach to the lateral surface of the thyroid cartilage of the larynx.	To retract the hyoid bone, the tongue, and the larynx. Both the tongue and larynx are attached to the hyoid bone and move as a unit.	Muscular branches of the common carotid artery. Ventral branches of the first and second cervical nerve

*The figures of these muscles are shown with muscles of neck in chapter-10

9

Muscles of Eyeball

Site of Incision

Make an incision around the eyeball at the margin of orbit.Then remove the supraorbital process by cutting dorsal and ventral end to access inside the orbit. Remove all the attachments of eyeball from osseous orbit through carefull dissection. Then remove all the extraoccular and periorbital fat to expose the muscles of eyeball.

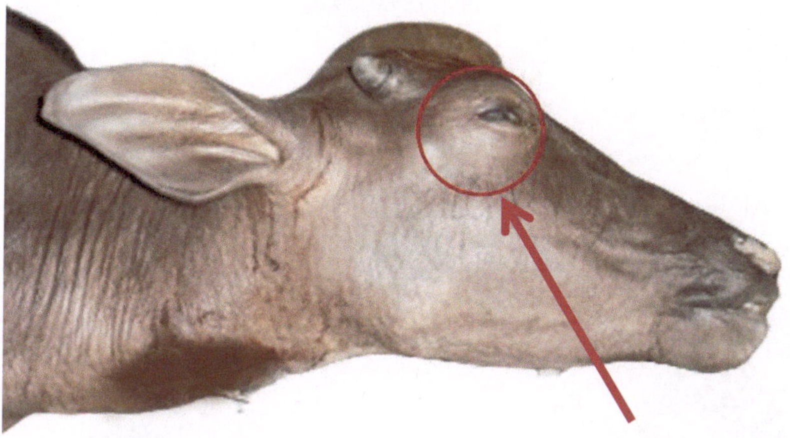

Fig. 9.1: Site of Incision (Arrow)

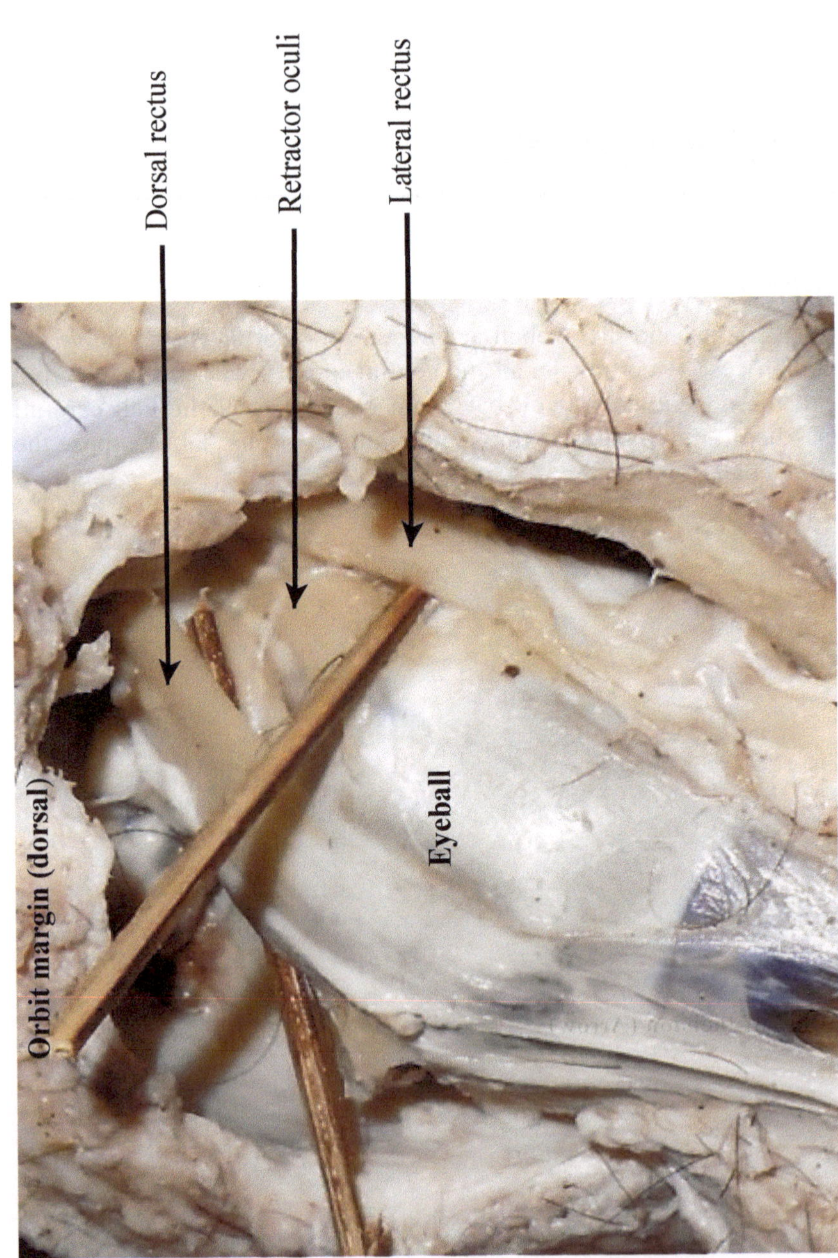

Fig. 9.2: Muscles of Eyeball

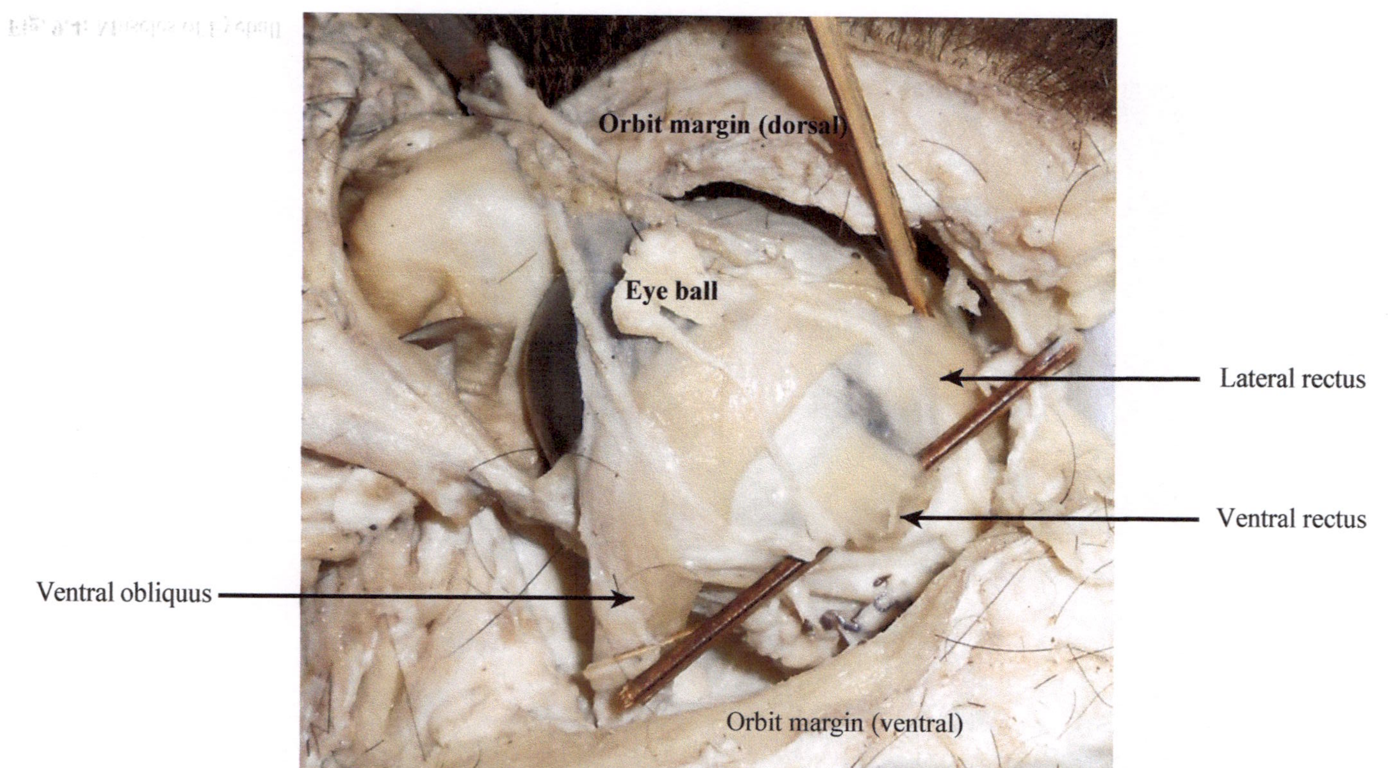

Fig. 9.3: Muscles of Eyeball

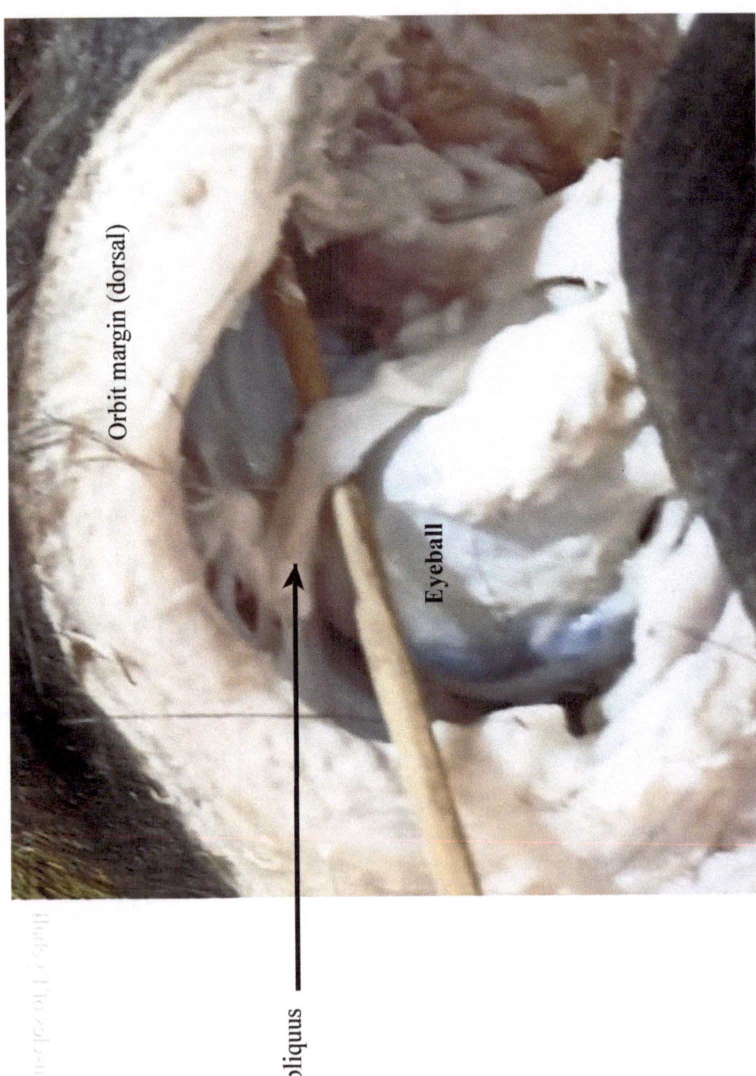

Fig. 9.4: Muscles of Eyeball

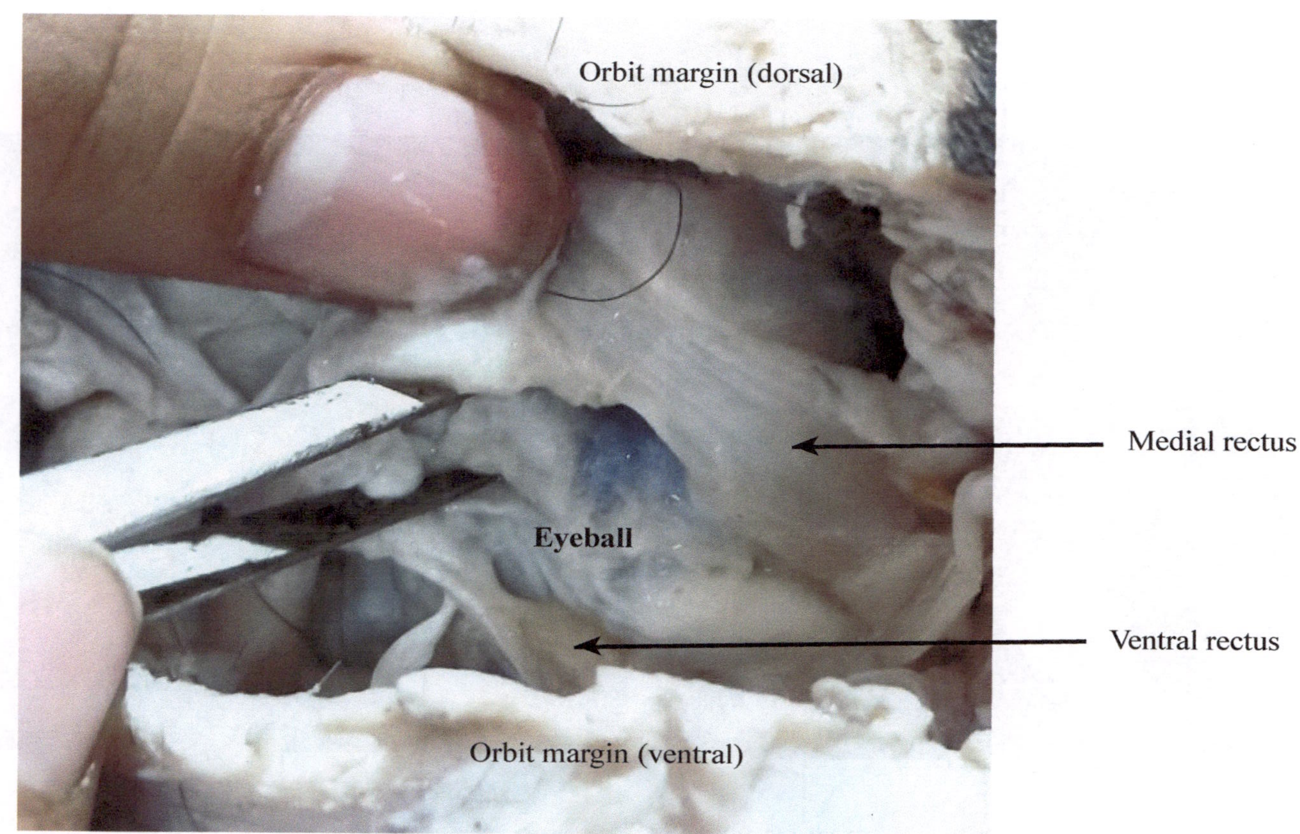

Fig. 9.5: Muscles of Eyeball

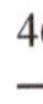

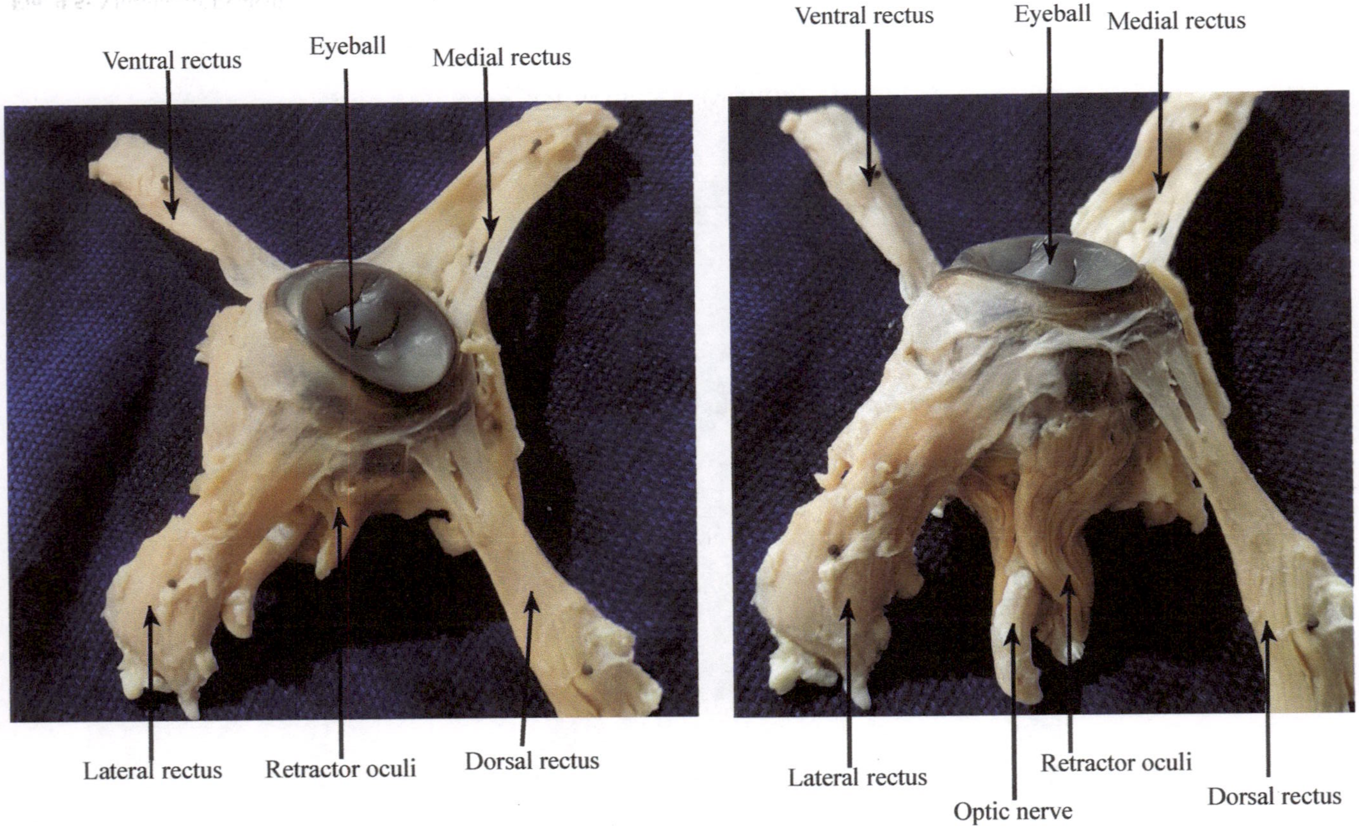

Fig. 9.6: Muscles of Eyeball (after removal from the orbit)

Table 9.1: Detail of Muscles of Eyeball

S.N	Name of muscle	Origin	Insertion	Action	Blood and Nerve supply
1.	Dorsal rectus	Around optic foramen	Inserted into sclera anterior to equator of eye	Rotate the eyeball about a transverse axis, moving the vertex of cornea dorsally and ventrally, respectively	Opthalmic artery Occulomotor nerve
2.	Ventral rectus	Around optic foramen	Inserted into sclera anterior to equator of eye	As above	Opthalmic artery Occulomotor nerve
3.	Medial rectus	Around optic foramen	Inserted into sclera anterior to equator of eye	Rotate the eyeball about vertical axis, moving the vertex of cornea medial and lateral, respectively	Opthalmic artery Occulomotor nerve
4.	Lateral rectus	Around optic foramen	Inserted into sclera anterior to equator of eye	As above	Opthalmic artery Abducens nerve
5.	Retractor oculi/ Retractor bulbi	Around optic foramen	Inserted into sclera posterior to recti	Draw the eyeball caudally and its parts may separately reinforce corresponding recti	Opthalmic artery Abducens nerve
6.	Dorsal obliquus	Near ethmoid foramen	Into sclera between dorsal and lateral recti, behind the margin of cornea.	Rotate the eyeball about a longitudinal axis, raises the lateral end of pupil	Opthalmic artery Trochlear nerve
7.	Ventral obliquus	Medial wall of orbit in small depression (muscular fossa) caudal to lacrimal fossa	Sclera near ventral margin of lateral rectus	Rotate the eyeball about a longitudinal axis, lowers the lateral end of pupil	Opthalmic artery Occulomotor nerve

10

Muscles of Neck Region

Site of incision: Make a midventral incision on the neck from larynx up to thoracic inlet then make ventrodorsal incision from both ends of this incision up to mid dorsal aspect of neck region.

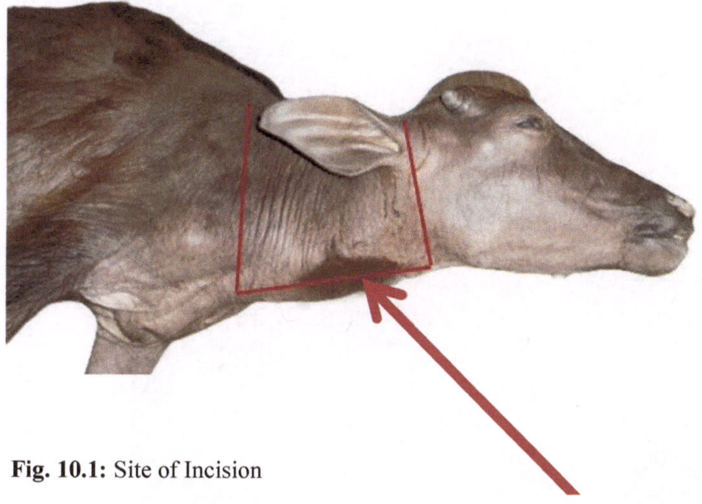

Fig. 10.1: Site of Incision

Ventral Cervical Muscles: This group of muscles are ventral to the cervical vertebrae

Laterodorsal Cervical Muscles: In this aspect the muscles are arranged in four layers. The muscles of first layer are trapezius cervicalis and in the second layer rhomboideus cervicalis, serratus cervicis and brachiocephalicus and omotransversarius. The splenius is in the third layer and Longissimus capitis et atlantis, Complexus, Multifidus cervicis, spinalis et semispinalis, longissimus cervicis, Obliquus capitis caudalis, Obliquus capitis cranialis, Rectus capitis dorsalis major, Rectus capitis dorsalis minor are in fourth layer.

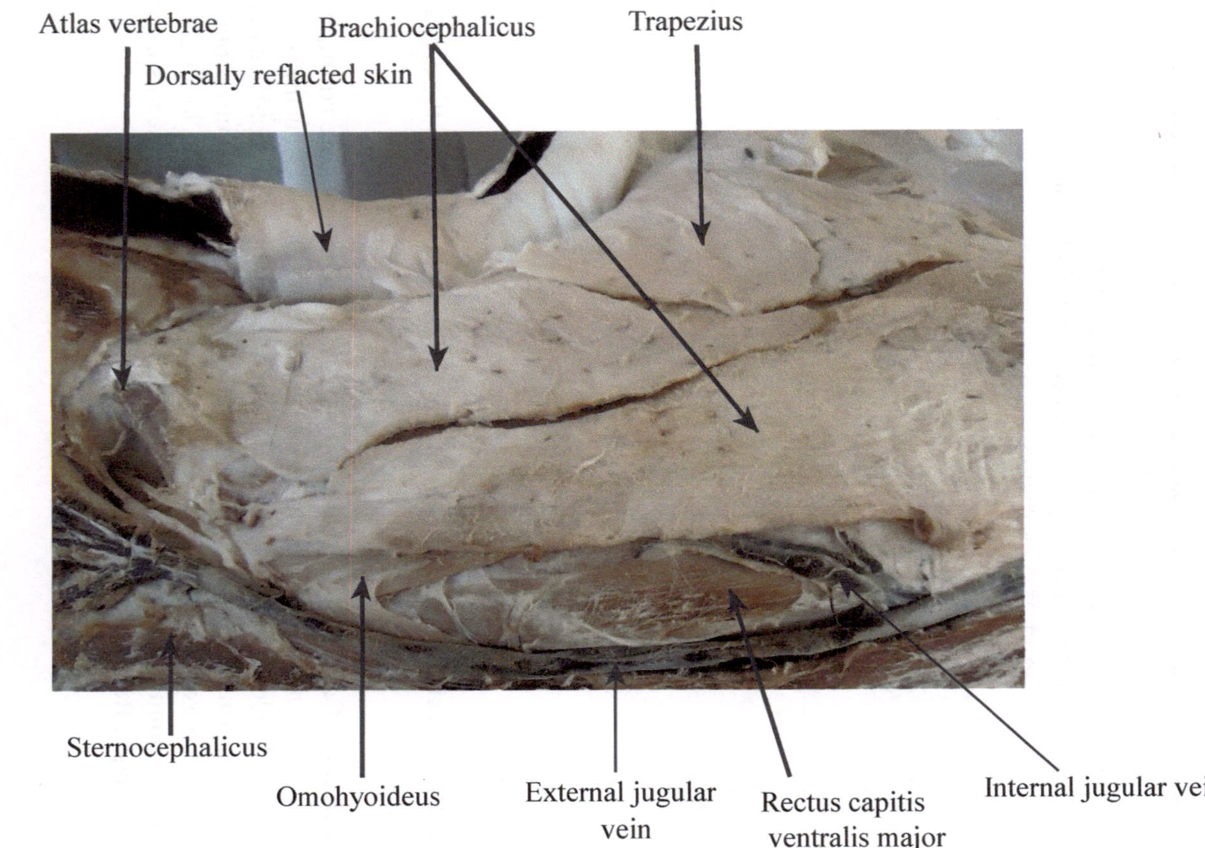

Fig. 10.2: Muscles of Neck Region: Ventral Cervical Group

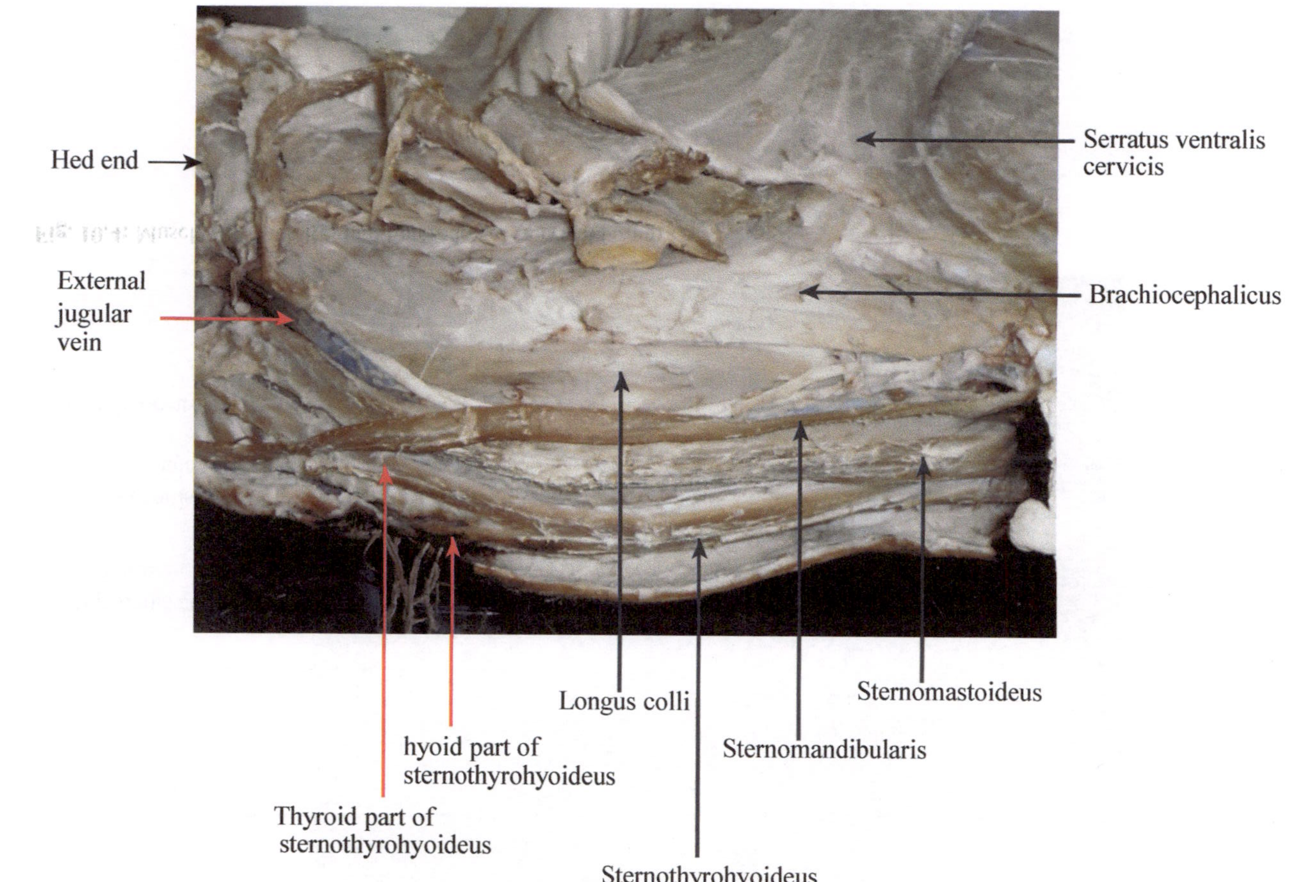

Fig. 10.3: Muscles of Neck Region: Ventral Cervical Group

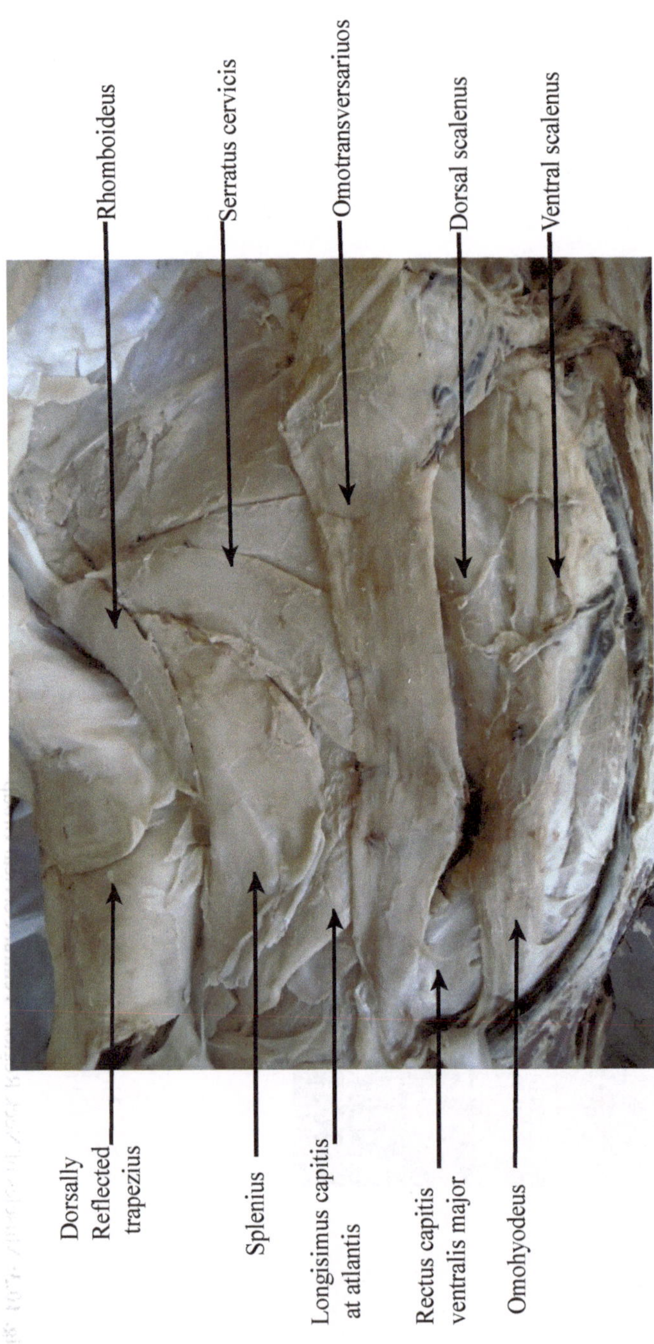

Fig. 10.4: Muscles of Neck Region: Laterodorsal Cervical Group

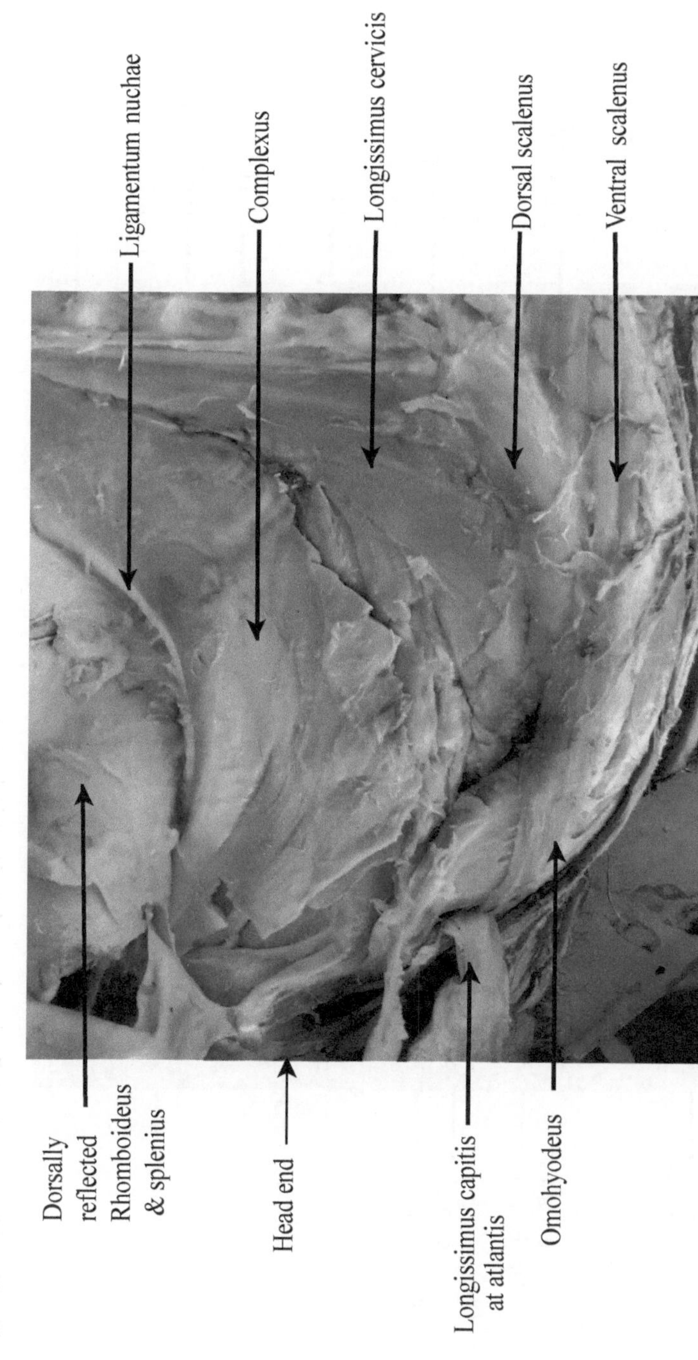

Fig. 10.5: Muscles of Neck Region: Laterodorsal Cervical Group

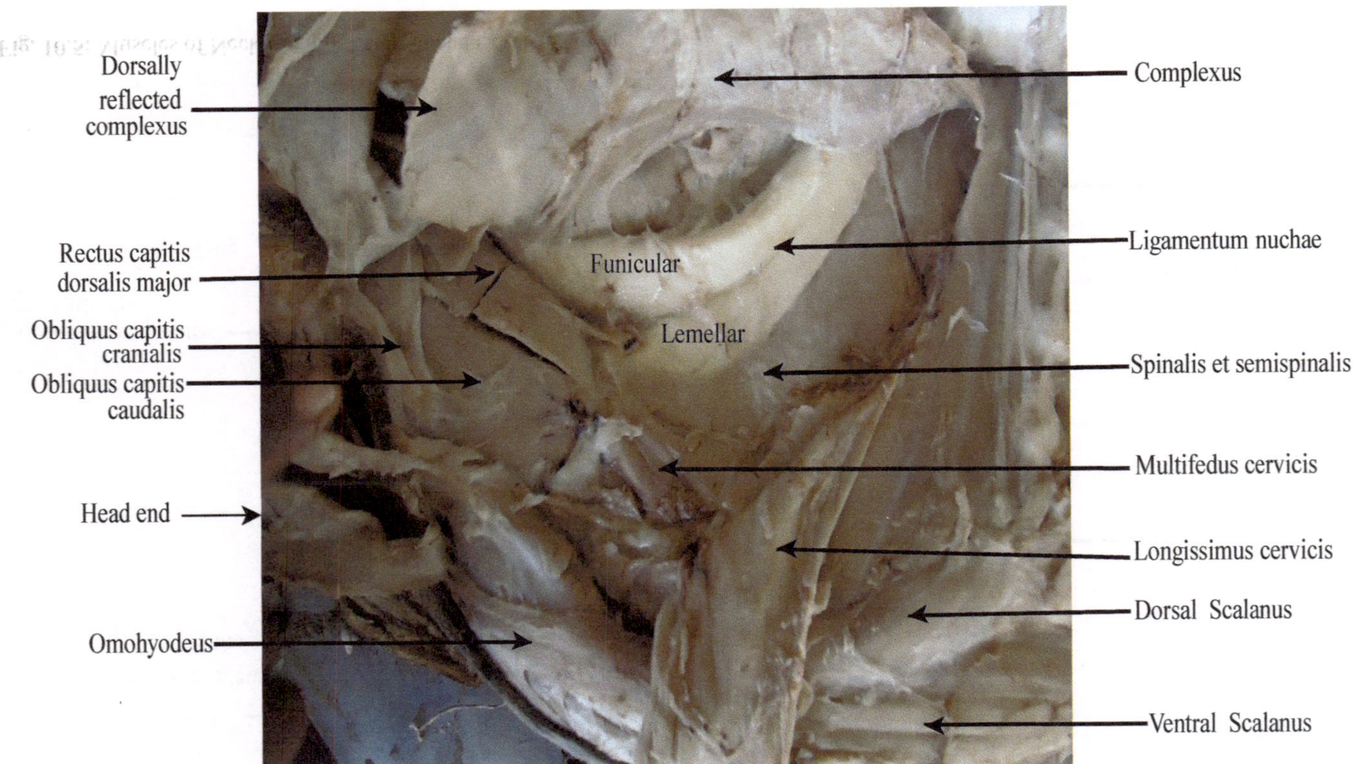

Fig. 10.6: Muscles of Neck Region: Laterodorsal Cervical Group

Table 10.1: Detail of Muscles of Ventral Cervical Group of Neck Region

S.N	Name of muscle	Origin	Insertion	Action	Blood and Nerve supply
1.	Sternocephalicus (mandibular part;sternomandibularis and mastoid part;sternomastoideus)	Both parts have their posterior attachment to manubrium sterni and the first costal cartilage.	Mandibular part inserts on the ventral border of the mandible and the fascia covering the masseter muscle. Mastoid part inserts on the mastoid process of the temporal bone.	Both parts flex the head on the neck and lower the head and neck. The mandibular part aids in opening the mouth by depressing the mandible. Some lateral flexion of the neck is also possible	Common carotid artery Ventral branch of the spinal accessory nerve
2.	Sternothyrohyoideus (Sternothyroideus and sternohyoideus part)	Anterior surface of the manubrium sterni.	The thyroid part, sternothyroideus, attaches to the lateral surface of the thyroid cartilage of the larynx. The hyoid part, sternohyoideus, inserts on the body of the hyoid bone.	To retract the hyoid bone, the tongue, and the larynx. Both the tongue and larynx are attached to the hyoid bone and move as a unit.	Muscular branches of the common carotid artery Ventral branches of the first and second cervical spinal nerve
3.	Scalenus a. Dorsal scalenus b. Ventral scalenus	a. Superficial part arise on transverse process of the sixth and possibly the fifth and fourth cervical vertebrae and deep part from transverse process of the seventh cervical vertebra b. Transverse processes of the fourth to the sixth cervical vertebrae	a. On the fourth rib and anterior border of the first rib, respectively. b. On the anterior border of the first rib.	Incline the neck laterally and to fix the first rib to inspiration. The superficial part may possibly aid inspiration.	Vertebral and inter costal arteries. Ventral branches of the cervical nerves.

S.N	Name of muscle	Origin	Insertion	Action	Blood and Nerve supply
4.	Rectus capitis ventralis major	Ventral branch of the transverse processes of the cervical vertebrae from the second to the sixth.	Basilar tubercle of occipital bone	Flex the head on the neck	Occipital and vertebral arteries Ventral branches of the cervical nerves from the second to the fifth.
5.	Rectus capitis ventralis minor	Ventral surface of the lateral mass of the atlas close to the posterior articular surface	Basilar tubercle of the occipital bone	To aid in flexing the head on the neck	Occipital artery Ventral branch of first cervical nerve
6.	Longus colli (Thoracic and cervial part)	Bodies of the first six thoracic vertebrae and the transverse processes of the cervical vertebrae except the atlas.	Thoracic part inserts on the bodies of the last two cervical vertebrae and the cervical part to the bodies of the cervical vertebrae and ventral tubercle of the atlas.	To flex the neck ventrally	Vertebral and subcostal arteries. The ventral branches of the cervical nerves except the first.
7.	Intertransversales colli (Each muscle has dorsal and ventral parts)	Origins and insertion are not recognized. It occupy the space between the articular and transverse processes on the lateral surface of the cervical vertebrae	Dorsal part extend from the upper part of the transverse process to the anterior articular process of the preceding vertebra. The ventral part extend between the ventral parts of the transverse processes.	To flex the neck laterally	Vertebral artery Ventral branches of the cervical nerves except the first and last.

Table 10.2: Detail of Muscles of Laterodorsal Cervical Group

S.N	Name of muscle	Origin	Insertion	Action	Blood and Nerve supply
1.	Trapezius (consist of 02 parts)				Dorsal branches of several inter costal arteries, the dorsal, deep cervical and posterior cervical arteries. Dorsal branch of the spinal accessory nerve
	A. Trapezius cervicalis	A fibrous raphae common to the right and left muscles extending from the first thoracic vertebra to the level of the axis.	The scapular spine by a narrow aponeurosis.	Lift the scapula upward.	
	B. Trapezius thoracic	Summits of the first six or seven thoracic spines	Tuber spine by a flat tendon		
2.	Rhomboideus (consist of 02 parts)			The cervical part pulls the upper part of scapula forward to inclines the neck and head laterally. The thoracic part draws scapula upward and a side in supporting the limb when it is in motion.	Dorsal and deep cervical arteries IV and VIII cervical nerves
	A. Rhomboideus cervicalis	From the level of the second thoracic to the second cervical vertebrae	Medial surface of the scapular cartilage		
	B. Rhomboideus thoracic	Summits of 2nd to 5th thoracic spines	Medial surface of the scapular cartilage		
3	Serratus ventralis (consist of 02 parts)				Vertebral, deep cervical, dorsal and intercostal arteries. Long thoracic nerve
	A. Serratus cervicis	The transverse process of the last five or six cervical vertebrae and the lateral surface of the first three ribs	Anterior triangular area on the costal surface of the scapula	Acting in unison they raise the body between the limbs. Acting singly to eventually shift the weight to the opposite limb. The cervical attachment may aid in elevating the neck. The thoracic attachment aids in forced inspiration	
	B. Serratus thoracic	The lateral surface of the four to the nine ribs	The rough line at supero-posterior part of scapula and medial face of cartilage of the scapula		

S.N	Name of muscle	Origin	Insertion	Action	Blood and Nerve supply
4.	Brachiocephalicus	Occipital bone (nuchal line) and the mastoid process of the temporal bone.	Crest of the humerus below the deltoid tuberosity	Draws the limb forward or inclines the head and neck laterally. The occipital attachment possibly extends the head on the neck.	Posterior cervical, common carotid, vertebral, and the posterior circumflex humeral arteries. Ventral branches of the cervical nerves except the last two and the axillary's nerve.
5.	Omotransversarius	The wing of the atlas and occasionally from the tranverse process of the axis	The fascia of the shoulder and occasionally to the scapular spine	To draw the shoulder and limb forward to incline the neck and head laterally.	Posterior cerviacal, common carotid, vertebral, and the posterior circumflex humeral arteries. Ventral brancheas of the cervical nerves, except the last two and the axillary' nerve.
6.	Splenius	Summits of the first three or four thoracic spines and fibrous raphe common to the right and left muscles	Transverse processes of the first three cervical vertebrae, the occipital bone with the cleido-occipitalis and the mastoid process of the temporal bone with the longissimus capitis muscle.	Elevate the head and neck and extend the head on the neck. Acting singly to incline the head and neck to the side of the muscle acting.	Deep cervical and to a small extent by the dorsal artery. Dorsal branches of the cervical spinal nerves except the first two.
7.	Longissimus capitis et atlantis	Transverse processes of the first two thoracic and the articular processes of cervical vertebrae except the first two or three	Atlantal part attaches to the posterior part of the lateral border of the atlas. Capitis part has a flat tendon that attaches to the mastoid process above the insertion of cleidomastoideus.	The atlantal part inclines the neck to the side of the muscle acting. Capitis part assists in extending the head on the neck.	Vertebral and deep cervical arteries. Dorsal branches of the cervical nerves except the first two.

S.N	Name of muscle	Origin	Insertion	Action	Blood and Nerve supply
8.	Complexus	Transverse processes of the first ten thoracic and the articular processes of the last five cervical vertebrae.	Nuchal line of the occipital bone.	To extend the head on the neck.	The deep cervical artery Dorsal branches of the first and second thoracic nerves and the sixth and seventh cervical nerves
9.	Rectus capitis dorsalis major	Anterior border of the spine of axis	Occipital bone near the external occipital protuberance	To extend the head on the neck.	Occipital artery Dorsal branch of first cervical nerve.
10.	Rectus capitis dorsalis minor	Dorsal arch of the atlas.	Occipital bone between the external occipital protuberance and the foramen magnum	Extend the head on the neck	Occipital artery Dorsal branch of first cervical nerve
11.	Obliquus capitis caudalis/posterior	Lateral surface of the spine and the posterior articular process of the axis.	Dorsal surface of the wing of the atlas.	To rotate the atlas on the axis. The head moves with the atlas, hence this muscle is an indirect rotator of the head.	Vertebral artery Second cervical nerve
12.	Oblique capitis cranialis/anterior	Anterior border and ventral surface of wing of atlas.	Mastoid and Para mastoid processes.	To extend the head on the atlas.	Occipital artery First cervical nerve
13.	Multifidus cervicis	Posterior articular process of each vertebra except the first two.	Posterior border of the posterior articular process and the spine of the preceding vertebrae.	Acting together to extend the neck; acting singly to produce lateral flexion and rotation	Vertebral and deep cervical arteries. Dorsal branches of the cervical nerves, except the first and second.

Note: Spinalis et semispinalis, longissimus cervicis are the parts of longissimus dorsi and described with muscle of back and loin.

11

Muscles of Thorax Region

Site of incision: Make a midventral incision on the sternum from cranial to caudal than from both ends of this incision make cranial incisions along the caudal border of shoulder and arm region to mid dorsal aspect of back and along last rib to mid dorsal aspect of back, respectively. Reflect the skin flap from ventral aspect to mid dorsal region of back.

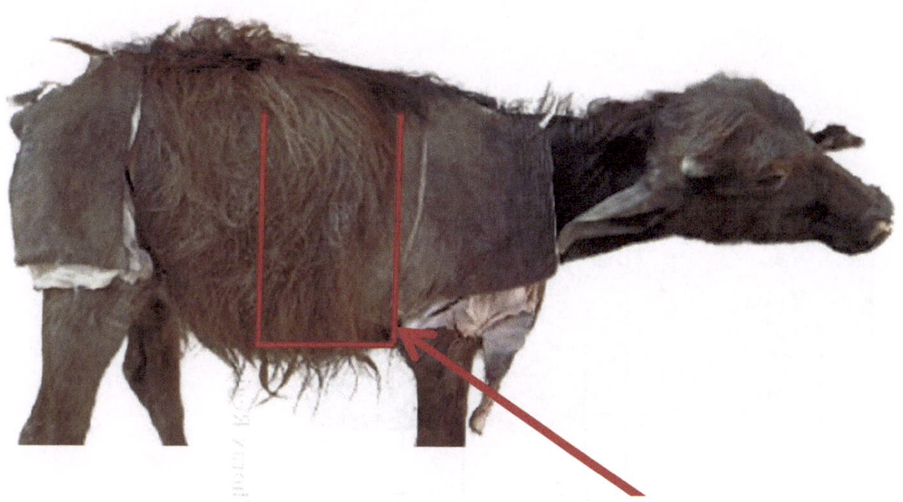

Fig. 11.1: Site of Incision (Arrow)

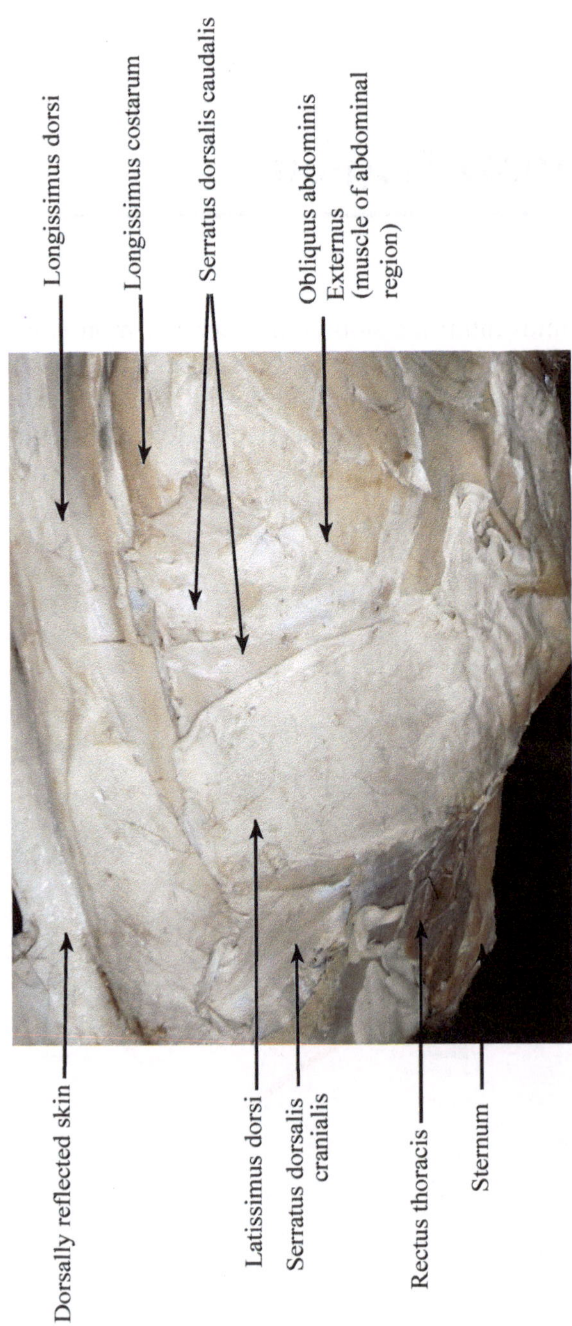

Fig. 11.2: Muscles of Thorax Region

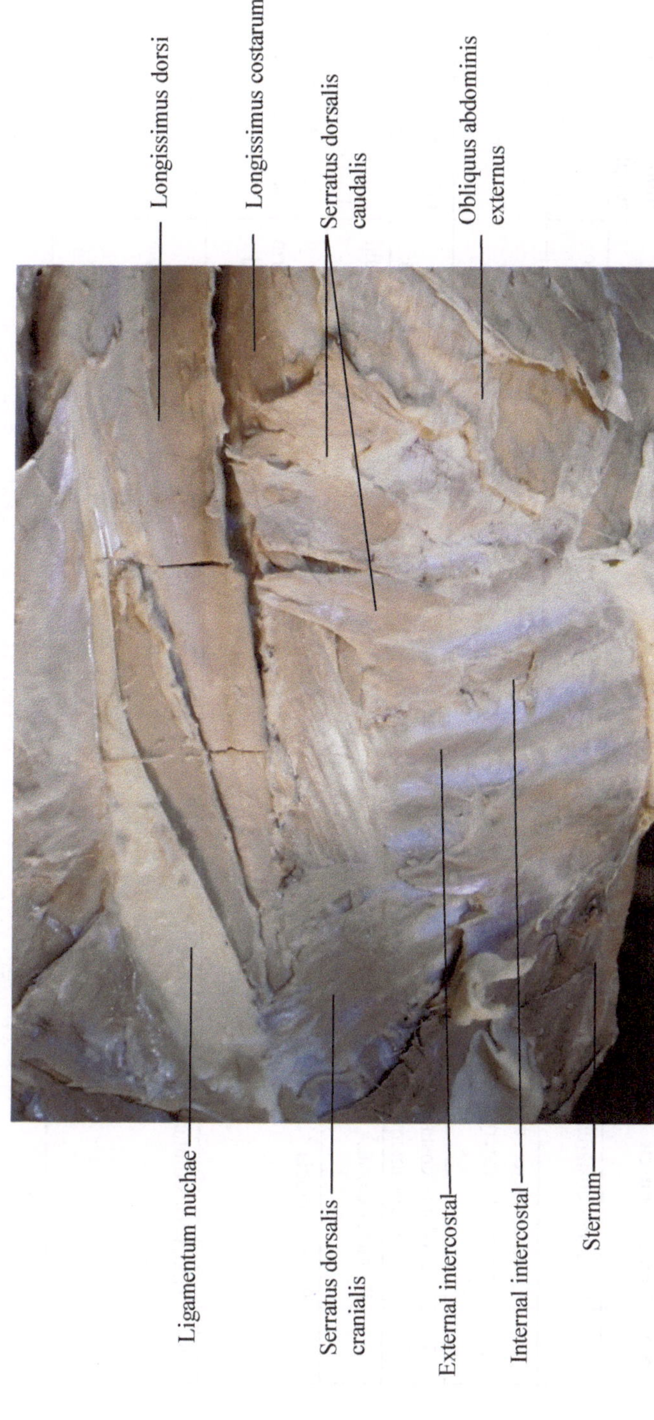

Fig. 11.3: Muscles of Thorax Region (after removal of Latissimus dorsi

Table 11.1: Detail of Muscles of Thorax Region

S.N	Name of muscle	Origin	Insertion	Action	Blood and Nerve supply
1.	Levatores costarum	Transverse processes of the thoracic vertebrae	Anterior border of the rib.	To draw the ribs forward to assist in inspiration.	Inter costal arteries and Inter costal nerves
2.	External intercostal/ Intercostalis externi	Posterior border of the rib	Anterior border of the succeeding rib.	To contract in sequence, drawing the ribs forward during inspiration.	Intercostal arteries Intercostal nerves
3.	Internal intercostal/ Intercostalis interni	Anterior border of the ribs except the first rib.	Posterior border of the preceding rib	To aid in expiration, especially forced expiration.	Intercostal arteries Intercostal nerves
4.	Retractor costae	Lumbodorsal fascia	Posterior border of the last rib	To retract the last rib and aid in forced expiration	Last intercostal artery .Last thoracic nerve
5.	Rectus thoracis	Ventral half of the first rib	Third or fourth costal cartilage	Assists in inspiration by drawing the cartilage and rib on which it inserts forward and outward.	Intercostal arteries Intercostal nerves
6.	Transversus thoracic	Sternal ligament	By digitations on the costal cartilages of the second to the sixth rib	Assist in expiration by drawing the costal cartilages and their ribs inward and backward.	Muscular branches of the internal thoracic artery. Second to sixth intercostal nerves.
7.	Diaphragm	It is a broad, unpaired muscle consist of a fleshy rim which may be subdivided into costal, sternal and a lumbar part; the lumbar part composed of two crura and a tendinous centre.			

Note:The muscle Serratus dorsalis is describe with muscles of back and loin region in chapter-12

12

Muscles of Back and Loin Region

Site of incision: Cut the skin over the back and loin region by making cranio-caudal straight incision along the proximal part of 1st rib and the lateral margin of transverse process of lumbar vertebrae up to wing of sacrum and reflect the skin to mid dorsal aspect of back and loin.

There are three layers of muscles in this region. The muscles of first layer are the trapezius thoracis (described with muscles of neck) and latissimus dorsi. The second layer consists of rhomboideus thoracis (described with muscles of neck), serratus dorsalis anterior and posterior. The muscles Longissimus costarum, Longissimus dorsi, Multifidus dorsi and Intertransversales lumborum are included in fourth layer.

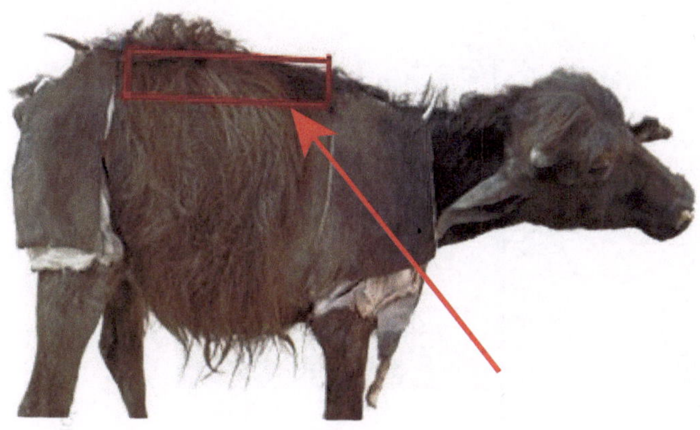

Fig. 12.1: Site of Incision (Arrow)

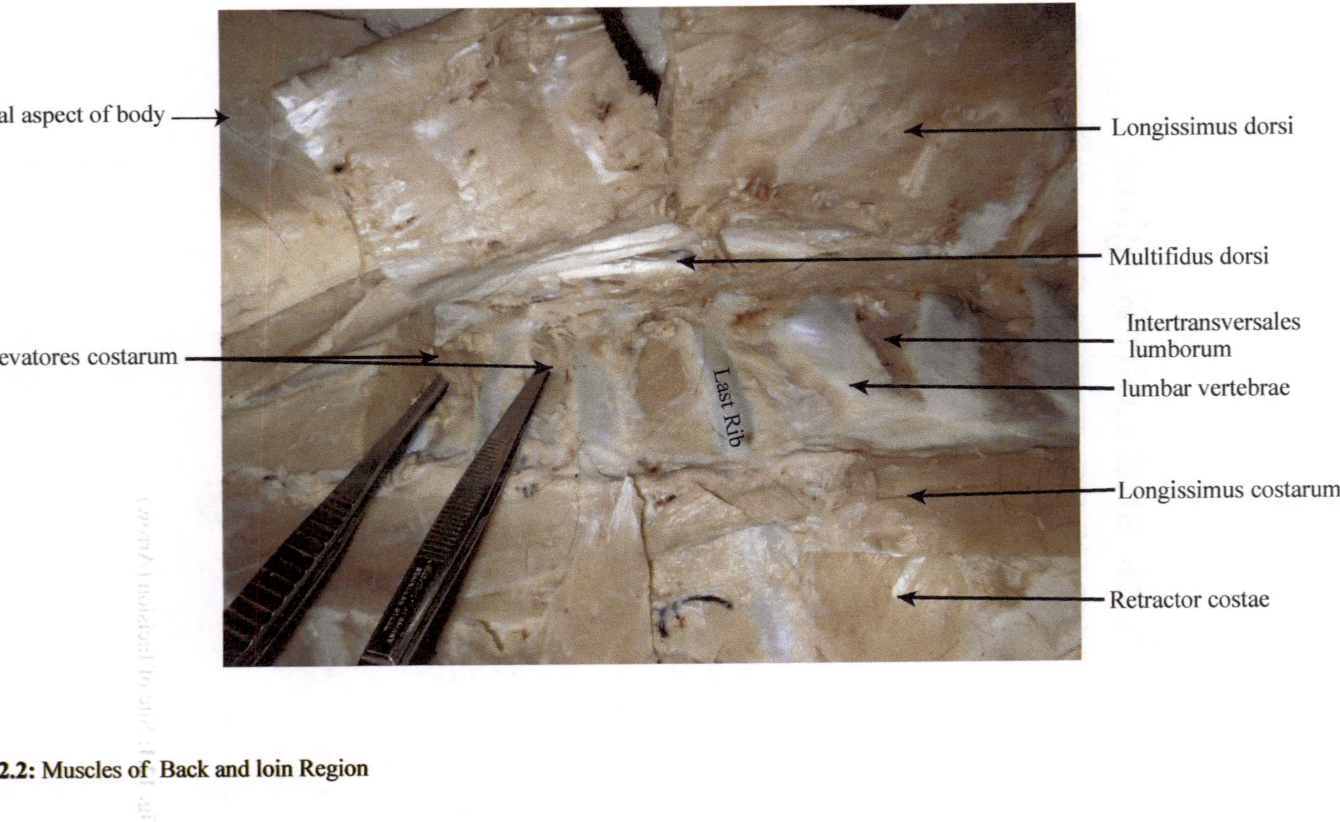

Fig. 12.2: Muscles of Back and loin Region

Table 12.1: Muscles of Back and Loin Region

S.N	Name of muscle	Origin	Insertion	Action	Blood and Nerve supply
1.	Latissimus dorsi	The superficial layers of the lumbodorsal fascia, from the fourth thoracic to the last lumbar spinous process	Teres tuberosity of humerus	This is reversible. When the limb is advanced and fixed, the body is drawn forward. When the limb is not supporting weight, it is drawn backward. The costal part may aid in inspiration.	Thoracodorsal, intercostal and lumbar arteries. Thoraco-dorsal nerve.
2.	Serratus dorsalis cranialis/anterior	By an aponeurosis detached from the deep layer of the lumbodorsal fascia.	Anterior border of six, seven, eight and nine rib	To aid in inspiration by drawing these ribs forward and outward.	Inter costal artery Thoracic nerves.
3.	Serratus dorsalis caudalis/posterior	Lumbodorsal fascia by a short aponeurosis.	Posterior border of the last three or four ribs.	To assist in expiration by drawing the ribs backward.	Inter-costal artery Thoracic nerves.
4.	Longissimus costarum	a. The lumbar portion from external angle of ilium b. The costal part arise from anterior border of last 8 or 9 ribs	a. The posterior border of last ribs b. Posterior border of ribs from 1st to 10th and to transverse process of last cervical vertebra	Chiefly to depress and retract the rib and help in expiration	Inter costal arteries Thoracic nerves.

5.	Longissimus dorsi*	Sacral spines, crest and adjacent part of ventral surface of the ilium, the lumbar spines through the lumbodorsal ligament and the thoracic spines	The transverse processes of the lumbar, thoracic and last three or four cervical vertebrae, the upper parts of the ribs and the spinous processes of the last three or four cervical vertebrae.	Most powerful extensor of the back, lateral flexion on the side of the contracting muscle is produced, The insertion to the cervical vertebrae tends to elevate the neck.	Lumbar arteries, dorsal branches of the intercostal arteries and the deep cervical artery. Dorsal branches of the lumbar, thoracic and cervical spinal nerves.
6.	Multifidus dorsi	Articular processes of the lumbar and transverse processes of the thoracic vertebrae.	The posterior border of the spinous processes of the first four lumbar and all of the thoracic vertebrae	Aid in extending the back. Acting on one side they flex the back laterally.	Intercostal and lumbar arteries. Dorsal branches of the thoracic and lumbar nerves.
7.	Intertransversales lumborum	A series of thin muscles occupying the spaces between the transverse processes of lumbar vertebrae except 5th and 6th.	The borders of adjacent processes	Aid in lateral flexion of the loin region.	Lumbar arteries Lumbar nerves

*This muscle is extends from the middle of the neck to the sacrum and ilium. In neck region it divides into two parts- 1. Longissimus cervicis (lateral part) 2. Spinalis et. Spinalis (medial part). The **longissimus cervicis muscle** has its origin from the transverse processes of the first six or seven thoracic vertebrae and insert to the transverse processes of last three or four cervical vertebrae. **spinalis et semispinalis muscle** lies, for the most part, against the thoracic spines and inserts on the spines of the last three or four cervical vertebrae.

13

Muscles of the Abdominal Region

Site of incision: Make a dorsoventral incision along caudal border of last rib up to mid ventral region of abdomen and another incision along the coxal tuber up to mid ventral region of abdomen. Joins the above two incision mid ventrally and reflect the skin up to mid dorsal aspect of lumber region.

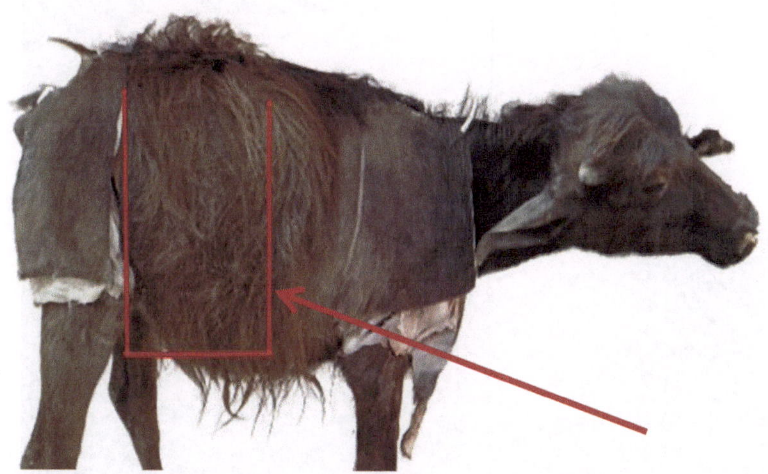

Fig. 13.1: Site of Incision (Arrow)

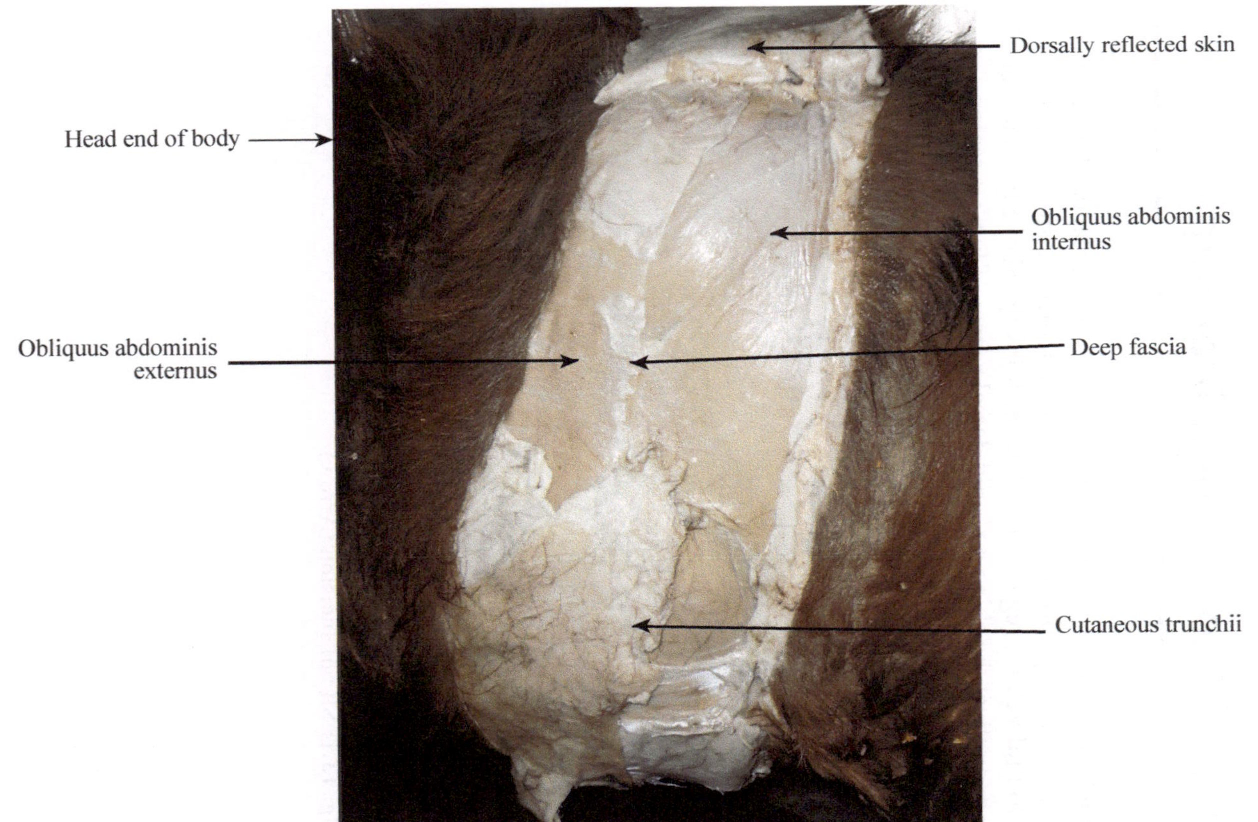

Fig. 13.2: Muscles of the Abdominal Region

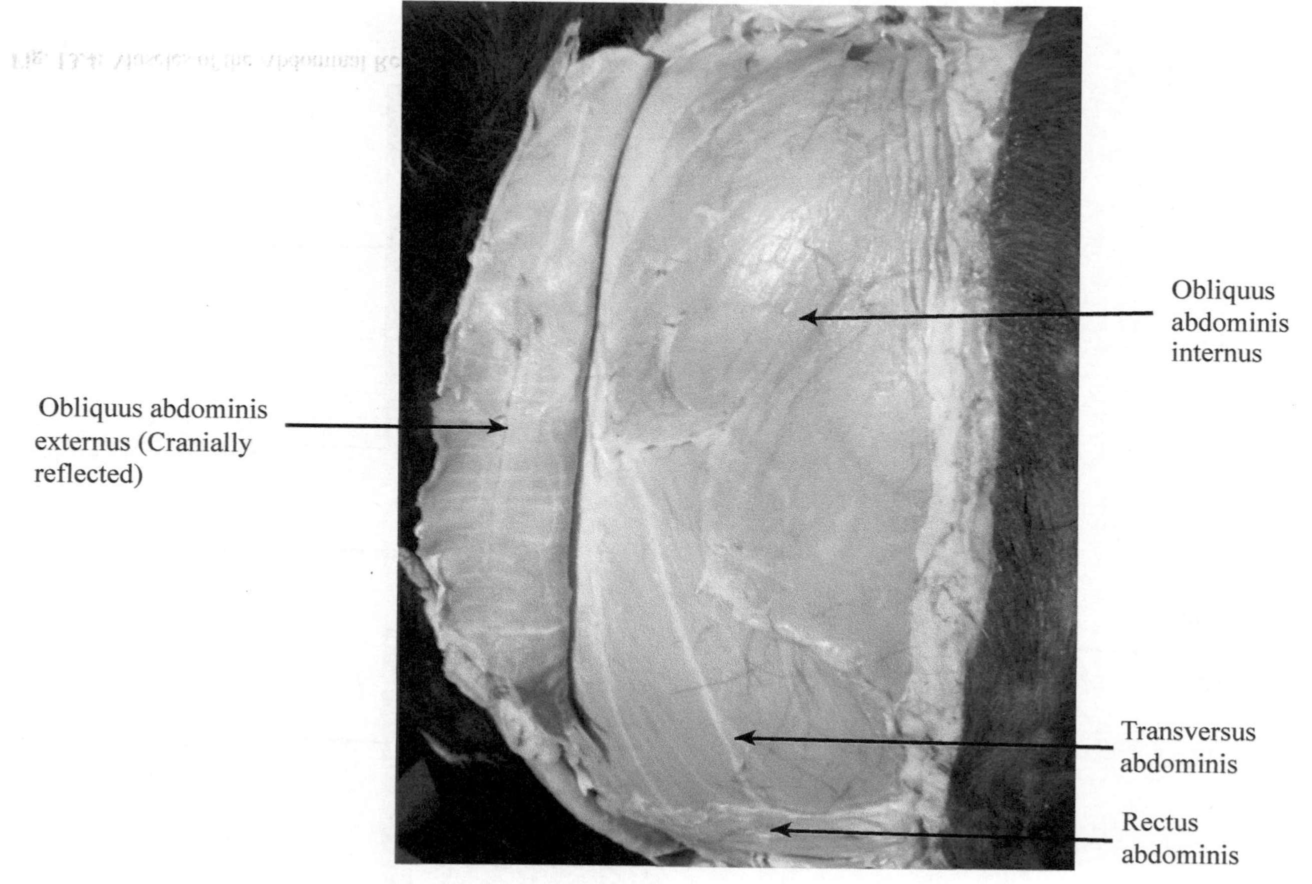

Fig. 13.3: Muscles of the Abdominal Region

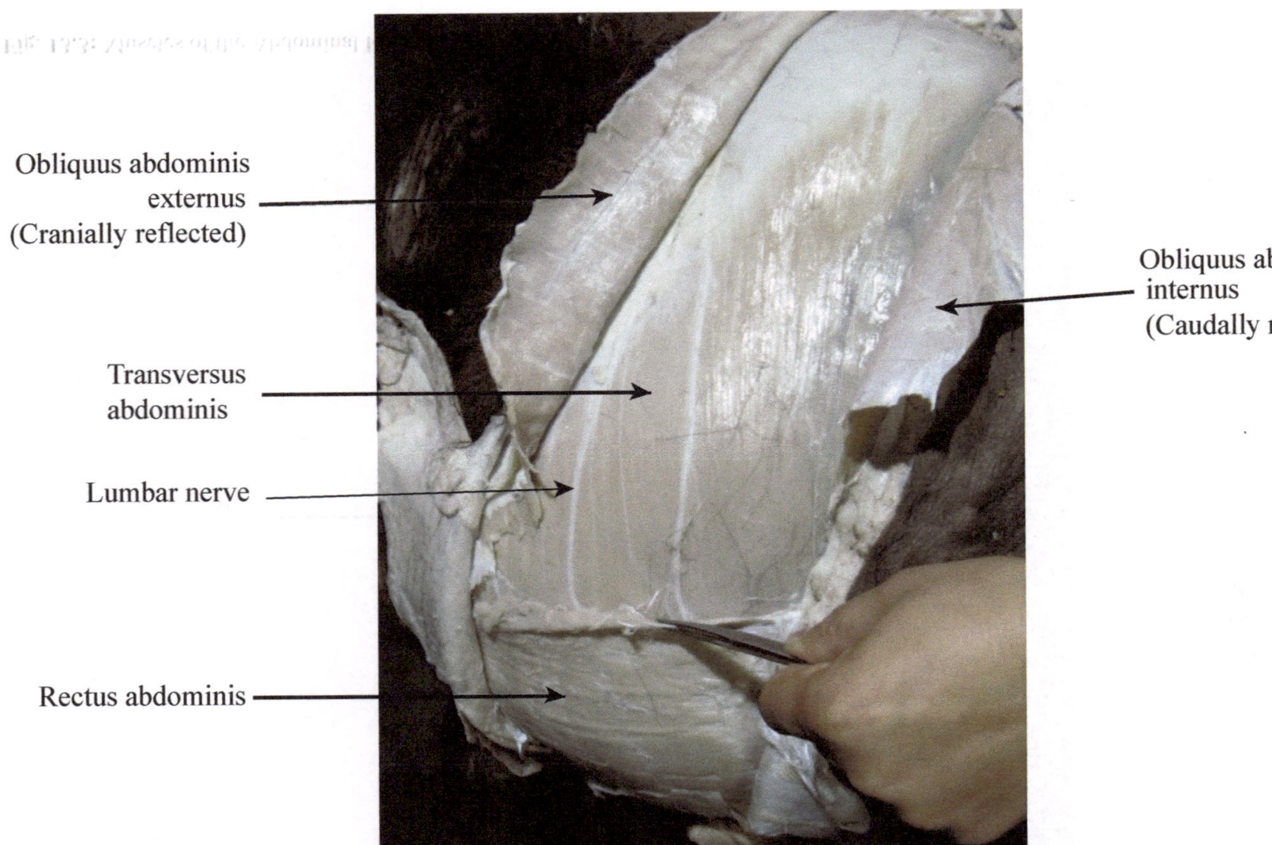

Fig. 13.4: Muscles of the Abdominal Region

Table 13.1: Detail of Muscles of the Abdominal Region

S.N	Name of muscle	Origin	Insertion	Action	Blood and Nerve supply
1.	External oblique muscle (Obliquus abdominis externus)	Posterior border and lateral surface of the last eight or nine ribs and the fascia covering the intervening intercostal muscles.	Tuber coxae, prepubic tendon, and linea alba. The entire insertion is aponeurotic	1. Compress the abdominal viscera, as in defecation micturition, parturition and expiration 2. Flex the trunk	The circumflex iliac and last intercostal artery Muscular branches of the first two lumbar and the last five or six intercostal nerves
2.	Internal oblique muscle (Obliquus abdominis internus)	Tuber coxae and the deep lumbar fascia at the lateral border of the longissimus dorsi.	Ventral half of the posterior border of the last rib and the ventral part of the prepubic tendon and the linea alba.	Same as above	The circumflex iliac, the posterior abdominal and last intercostal artery. Deep branches of the first two lumbar and the last thoracic nerves
3.	Transversus abdominis	Deep lumbar fascia and by this from the extremities of the first four lumbar transverse processes and the medial surface of the asternal ribs.	Linea alba and Xyphoid cartilage	Same as above	Anterior branch of the circumflex iliac, musculophrenic and intercostal arteries. The first two lumbar nerves and the last seven or eight intercostal nerves.
4.	Rectus abdominis	Ventral and lateral surfaces of the sternum as far forward as the third costal cartilage	Pecten pubis by means of the prepubic tendon	In addition to above actions it is especially adapted to flex the lumbosacral joints and the lumb and thoracic parts of the spine	Anterior and posterior abdominal arteries. The last six or seven thoracic and the first two or three lumbar nerves

14

Muscles of Sublumbar Region

Site of incision: Remove the abdominal viscera to expose the sublumber region.

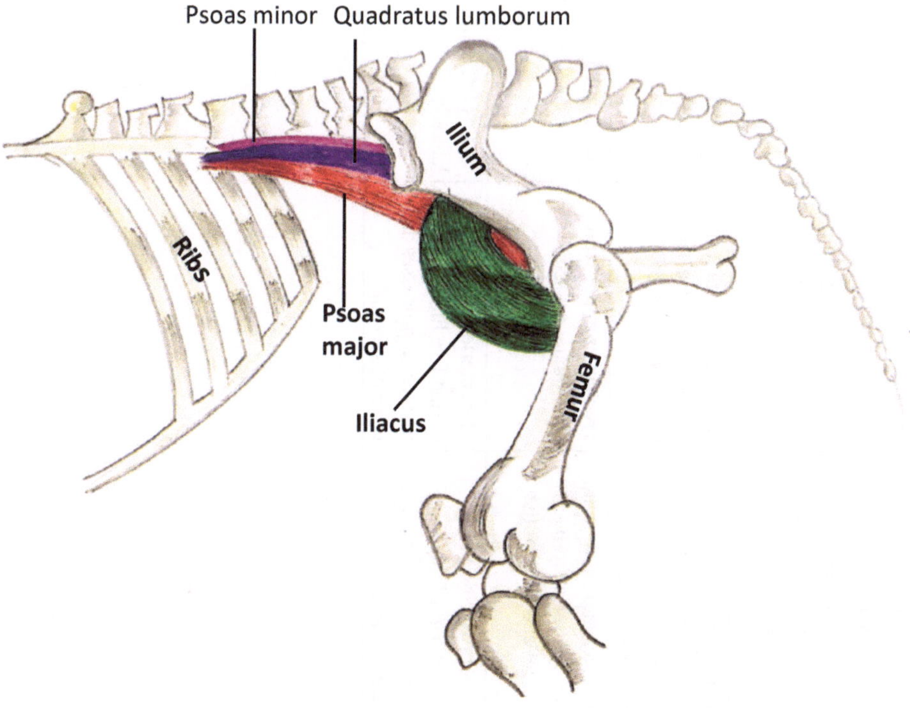

Fig.14.1: Muscles of Sublumbar Region

Table 14.1: Detail of Muscles of Sublumbar Region

S.N	Name of muscle	Origin	Insertion	Action	Blood and Nerve supply
1.	Psoas minor	The lateral surface of the bodies of the last thoracic and all lumbar vertebrae	Psoas tubercle on the shaft of the ilium	Flex the lumbo sacral joint and aid in arching the back	Branches from the lumbar arteries. Ventral branches of the lumbar nerves.
2.	Psoas major	The upper part of the last one or two ribs and the transverse processes of lumbar vertebrae.	The trochanter minor by a tendon which also serves the iliacus muscle	To flex the hip joint and to rotate the thigh outward.	Lumbar and circumflex iliac arteries. Lumbar nerves and iliopsoas branch of the femoral nerve.
3.	Iliacus	Pars iliaca and shaft of the ilium, ventral sacroiliac ligament and wing of the sacrum	Trochanter minor with psoas major muscle	To flex the hip joint and to rotate the thigh outward.	Ilio lumbar and deep femoral arteries. Iliopsoas branch of the femoral nerve and Lumbar nerves
4.	Quadratus lumborum	The last two ribs and adjacent part of the vertebrae and the first five lumbar transverse processes.	The anterior border of first five lumbar transverse processes and wing of sacrum	To flex the lumbar region laterally	Lumbar arteries Lumbar nerves

15

Muscles of Penis

Site of incision: Make a transverse incision below the anus between lateral margins of tuber ischia. Then from each end of this incision make an oblique incision caudo-cranially so that these join midventrally each other between the thighs. Remove the triangular flap of skin to expose the region.

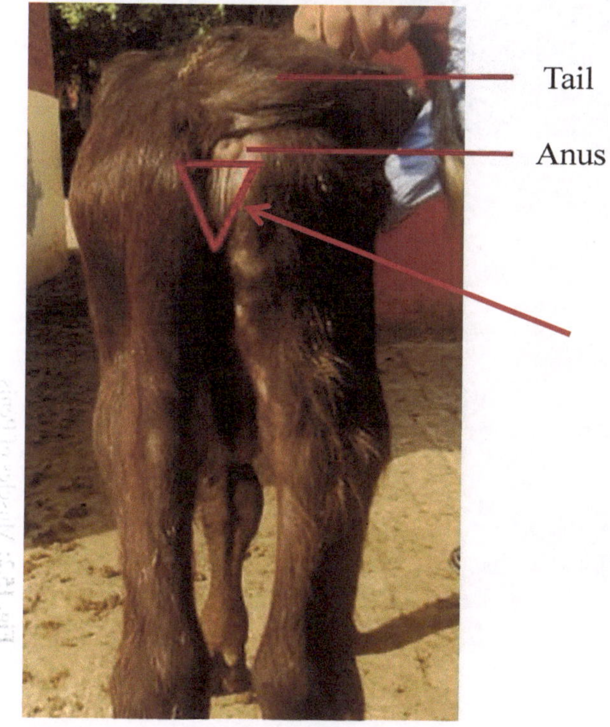

Fig. 15.1: Site of Incision (Arrow)

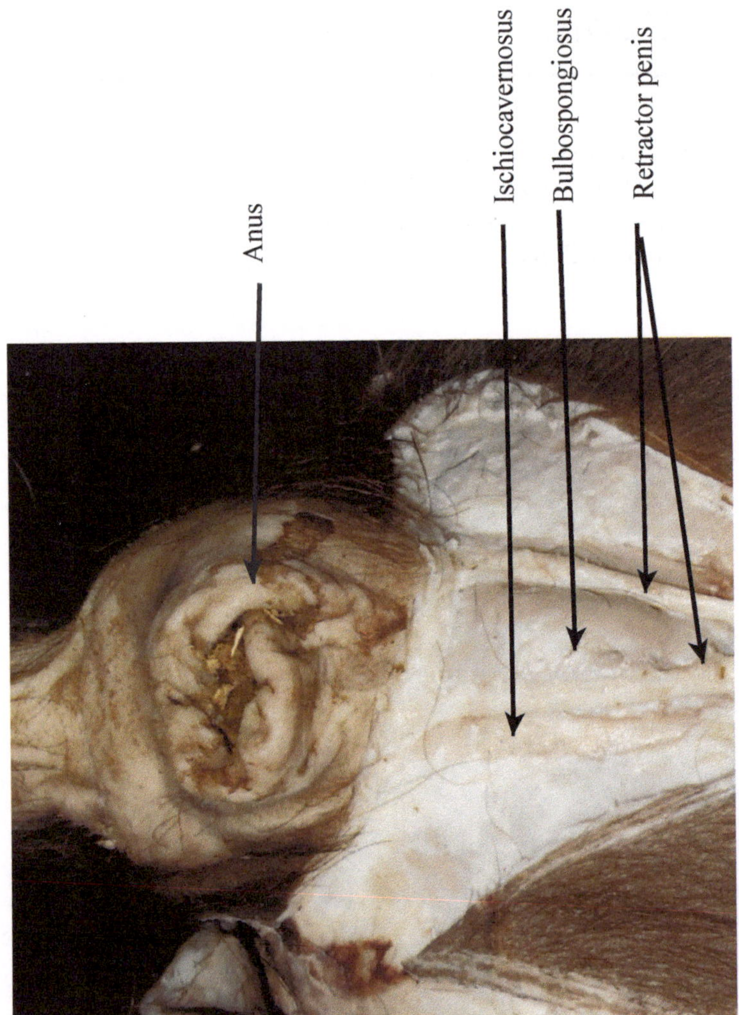

Fig. 15.2: Muscles of Penis

Table 15.1: Detail of Muscles of Penis

S.N	Name of muscle	Origin	Insertion	Action	Blood and Nerve supply
1.	Ischiocavernosus	Tuber ischii and the adjacent part of the sacro-sciatic ligament	Crus and adjacent part of the body of the penis	Pulls the penis against the pelvis, and assists in producing and maintaining erection by compressing the dorsal veins of the penis	Artery of bulb and pudic nerves.
2.	Retractor penis	Ventral surface of the first and second coccygeal vertebrae	Insertion is to the penis at anterior to the ventral bend of the sigmoid flexure	Withdraw the penis into the sheath after erection or protrusion.	Perineal artery, artery of bulb and sympathetic fibers of pudic nerve
3.	Bulbo-cavernosus	Originate at pelvic outlet below the anus and extend downward and little forward for a distance of about eight inches on the posterior surface of the penis.		Compress the urethra.	Artery of bulb and pudic nerves

16

Muscles of Hip and Thigh Region (Lateral Aspect)

Site of incision: Make an incision from distal end of cranial margin of stifle joint to coxal tuber and extend it dorsally up to mid dorsal line of the body. Make another incision at mid caudal of thigh from stifle region to tuber ischii and extend it to mid dorsal up to the base of the tail and then connects the distal ends of both previous incisions and reflect the skin up to mid dorsal line of the body.

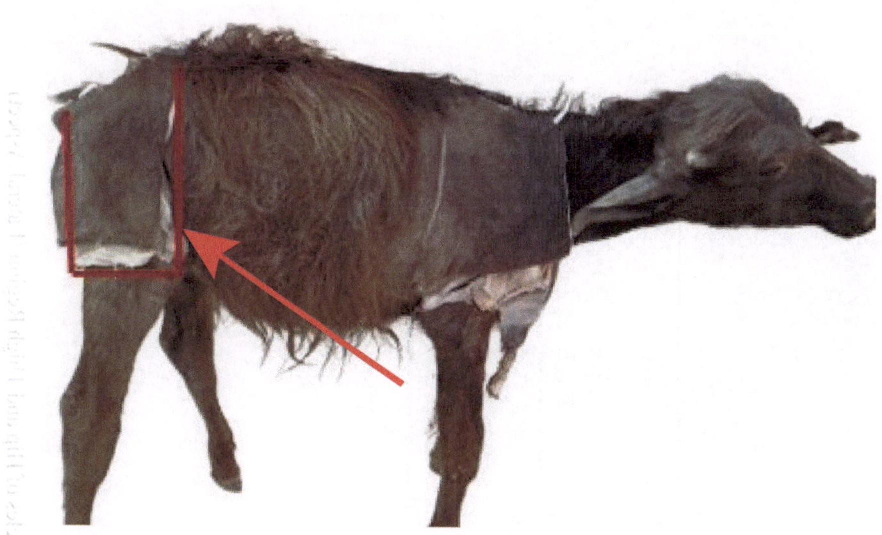

Fig. 16.1: Site of incision (Arrow)

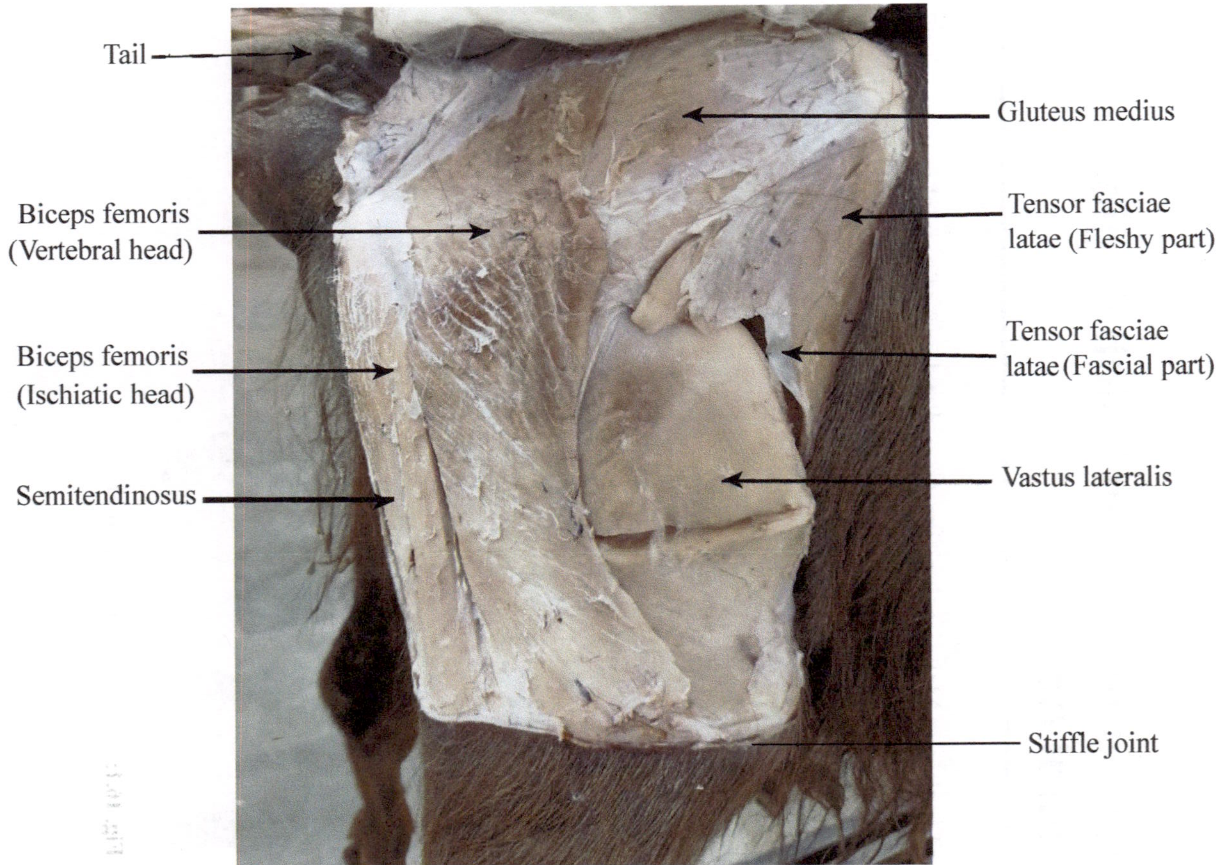

Fig.16.2: Muscles of Hip and Thigh Region (Lateral Aspect)

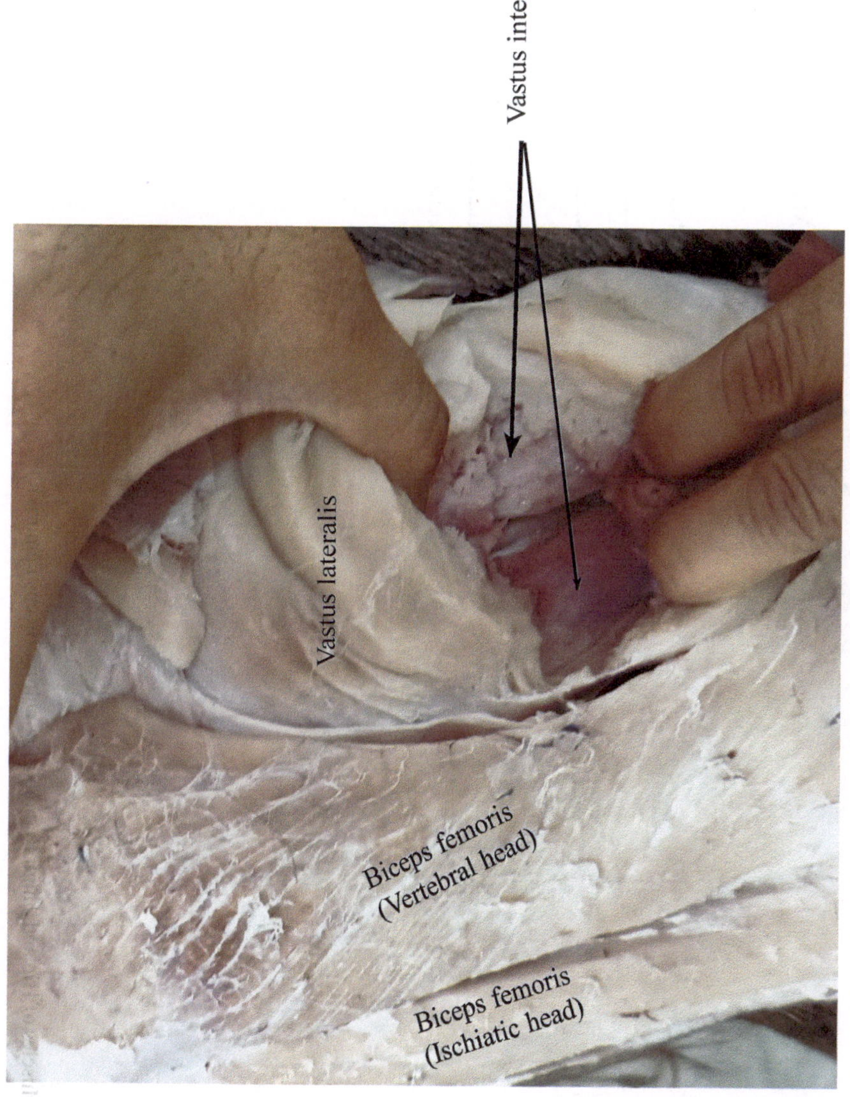

Fig.16.3: Muscles of Hip and Thigh Region (after cutting vastus lateralis)

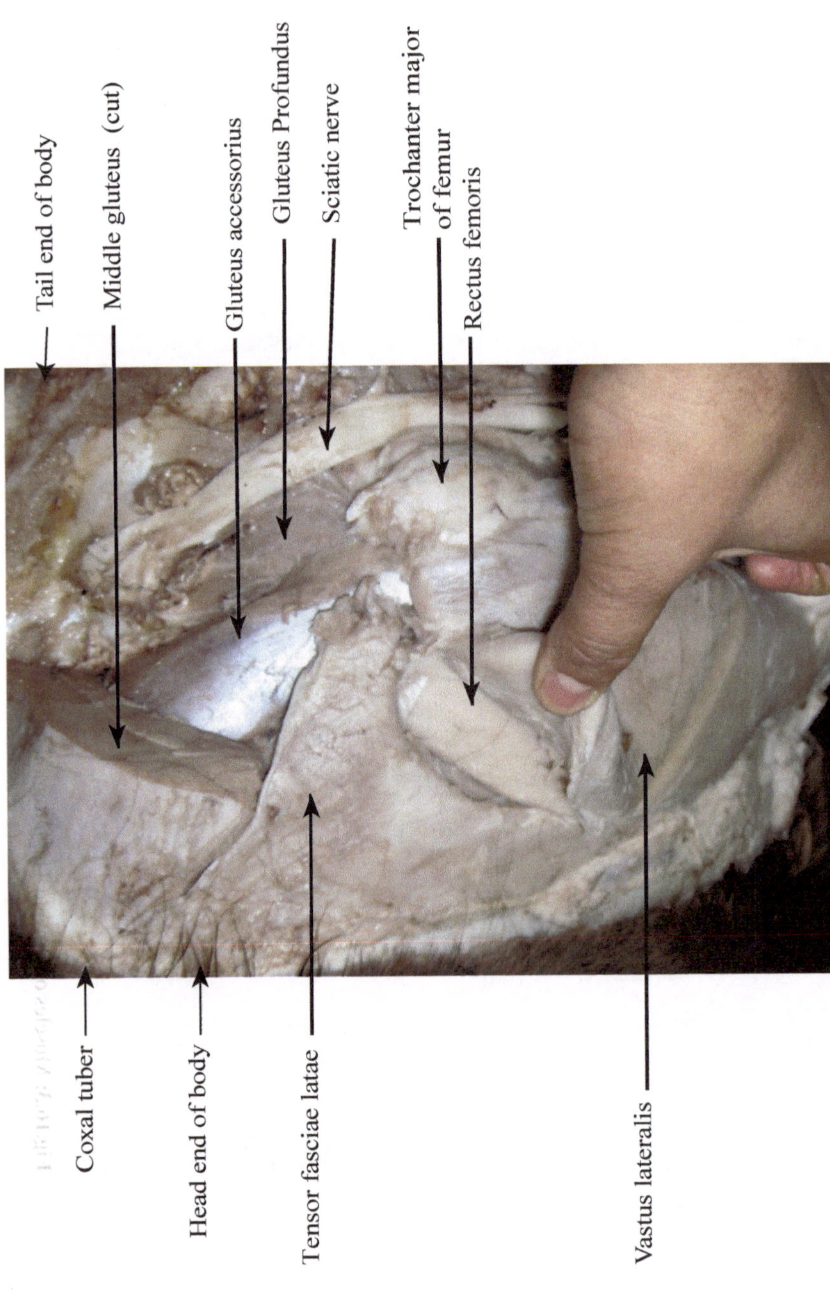

Fig.16.4: Muscles of Hip and Thigh Region (after cutting Biceps Femoris)

Table 16.1: Detail of Muscles of Hip and Thigh region (Lateral Aspect)

S.N	Name of muscle	Origin	Insertion	Action	Blood and Nerve supply
1.	Tensor fasciae latae (Facial part and fleshy part)	Tuber coxae and the deep gluteal fascia	Fascia lata and by this means to the patella. The latter is attached to the tibial tuberosity by patellar ligament.	Flex the hip and extend the stifle.	Posterior branch of the circumflex iliac artery. The long, lateral branch of the anterior gluteal nerve.
2.	Gluteus medius/ middle gluteus*	1. The aponeurosis of longissimus dorsi as far forward as the fifth lumbar vertebra. 2. Gluteal surface of ilium medial to the gluteal line 3.The tuber of the ilium, lateral sacro-iliac ligament	1.Free margin of the trochanter major, 2.Crest below trochanter 3. Lateral aspect of trochanteric ridge	Extend the hip joint, rotate the limb outward, abduct the limb and assist in rearing.	Anterior gluteal artery and posterior branch of the circumflex iliac artery Anterior gluteal nerve.
3.	Gluteus profundus	Lateral surface of the ischiatic spine, the gluteal line and sacrosciatic ligament.	A rough area just below the anterior margin of the trochanter major.	Rotate the anterior surface of the limb inward and flex the hip joint.	Anterior gluteal and anterior femoral arteries. Anterior gluteal nerve.
4.	Biceps femoris**	Lateral and dorsal sacroiliac ligaments, the posterior border of the sacrosciatic ligament, the lateral surface of the tuber ischii and fascia lata.	Patella, lateral patellar ligament, tibial crest and tuber calcis.	Extend the hip, stifle and hock joints in propulsion and kicking. The tibial attachment flex the stifle when the limb is not supporting weight. With the pelvic limbs stationary, it aids in rearing.	Anterior and posterior gluteal; deep femoral and posterior femoral arteries. Posterior gluteal and sciatic nerves.

S.N	Name of muscle	Origin	Insertion	Action	Blood and Nerve supply
5.	Semitendinosus	Lateral tuberosity of the tuber ischii.	A rough area on the medial surface of the tibial crest and the tuber calcis	Extend the hip, stifle and hock in walking and kicking. The tibial insertion flexes the stifle when the limb is being flexed. The action on the hip is indirect since there is no attachment to the femur. It assists in rearing and rotates the limb inward.	Deep femoral and posterior Femoral arteries Sciatic nerve.
6.	Quadriceps femoris Four Heads: (S.N. a-d)	All heads are attach to the patella and through the patellar ligaments to the tibial tuberosity.			Anterior femoral artery supplies all four heads. In addition, the vastus medialis received branches from the femoral artery. Femoral nerve
a	Rectus femoris	Shaft of the ilium by two tendons. The lateral tendon attaches in a depression above the acetabulum and the medial tendon in a depression anterior to the acetabulum.	Anterior part of the base of the patella.	Extend the stifle and flex the hip.	-
b	Vastus lateralis	Proximal two-thirds of the lateral surface of the femur and the lower part of the trochanter major.	Lateral border of the base of the patella on the lateral patellar ligament.	Extend the stifle joint	-

S.N	Name of muscle	Origin	Insertion	Action	Blood and Nerve supply
c	Vastus medialis***	The proximal two-thirds of the medial surface of the femur.	The medial border of the patella and the medial patellar ligament.	Extend the stifle joint	-
d	Vastus intermedius	The proximal two-thirds of the anterior surface of the femur.	The base of the patella behind the insertion of the rectus femoris.	Extend the stifle joint and raise the femoro-patellar capsule	-

*The pelvic portion of the muscle divided into superficial and deep part (**Gluteus accessorius**)

**The muscle has two head; the long or vertebral head and short or ischiatic head

***This is muscle of medial aspect of thigh

17

Muscles of Hip and Thigh Region (Medial Aspect)

Site of incision: Abduct the hind limb well apart and remove the skin covering the medial aspect of thigh. To obtain this make an incision longitudinally along the entire length of pelvic symphysis. From both ends of this incision make vertical incision up to medial aspect of stifle joint and joins distal end of these vertical incision together and remove the skin to expose the muscles of medial aspect of thigh region. To expose deeper muscles incise the vertebral attachment of biceps femoris, reflect it caudally by incising muscle close to stifle than reflect middle gluteus muscle dorsocranially and observe the deeper layer of muscles.

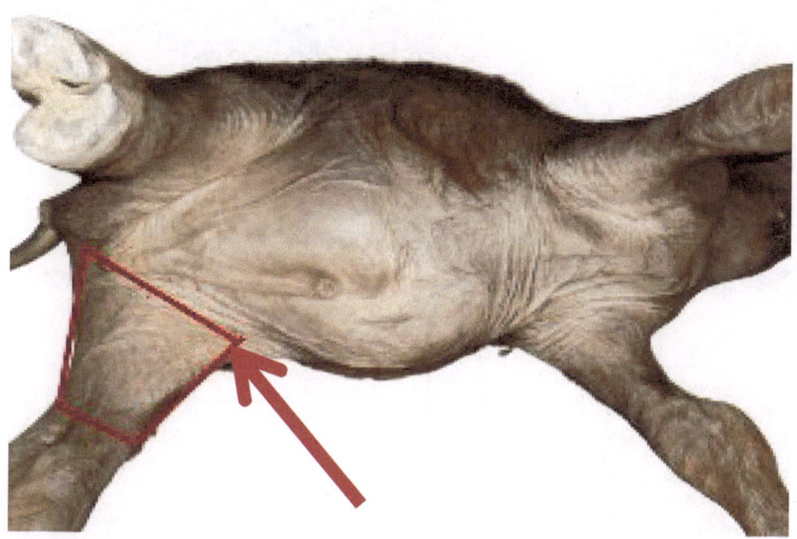

Fig. 17.1: Site of Incision (Arrow)

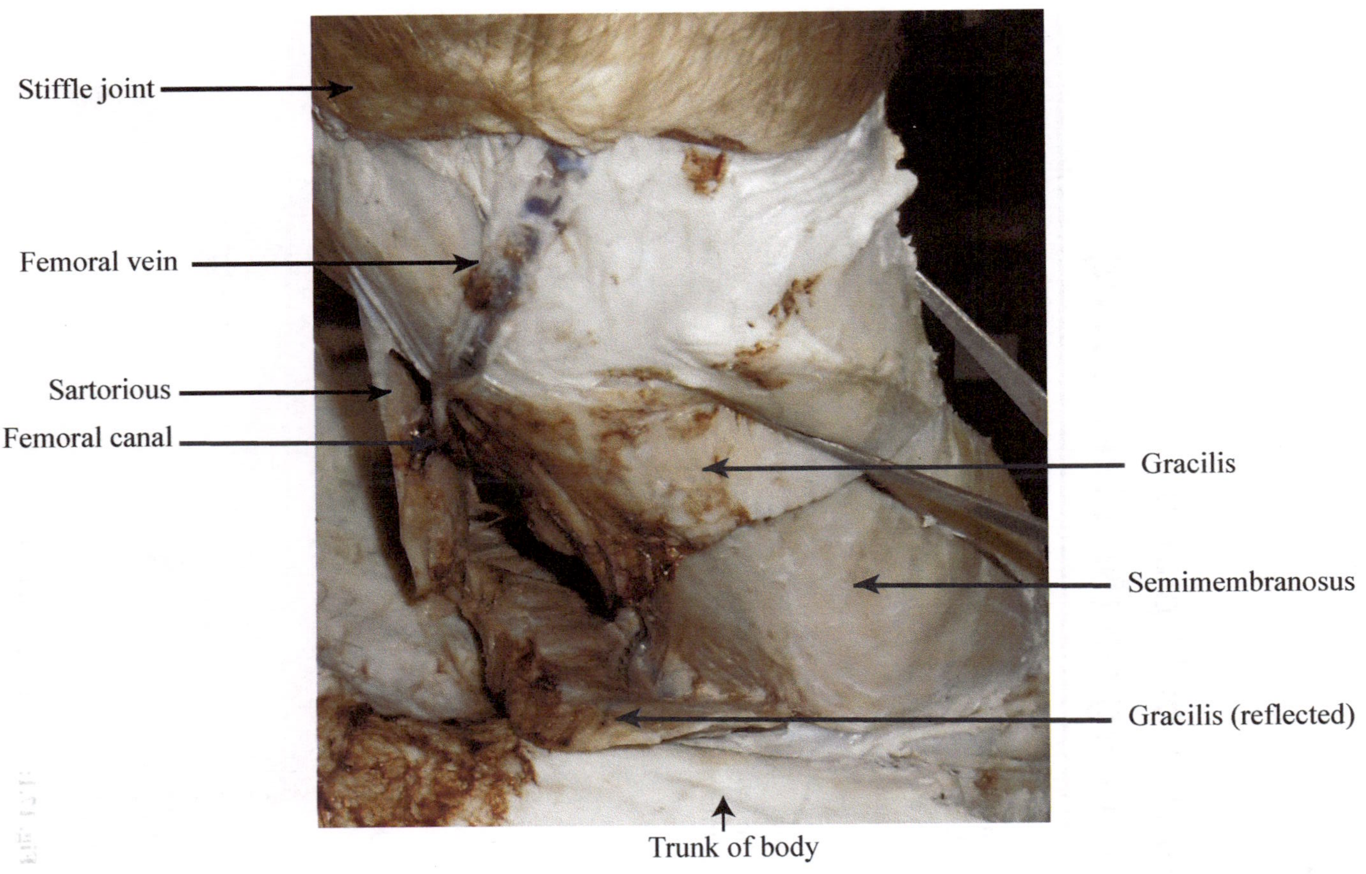

Fig. 17.2: Muscles of Hip and Thigh Region (Medial Aspect) after abduction

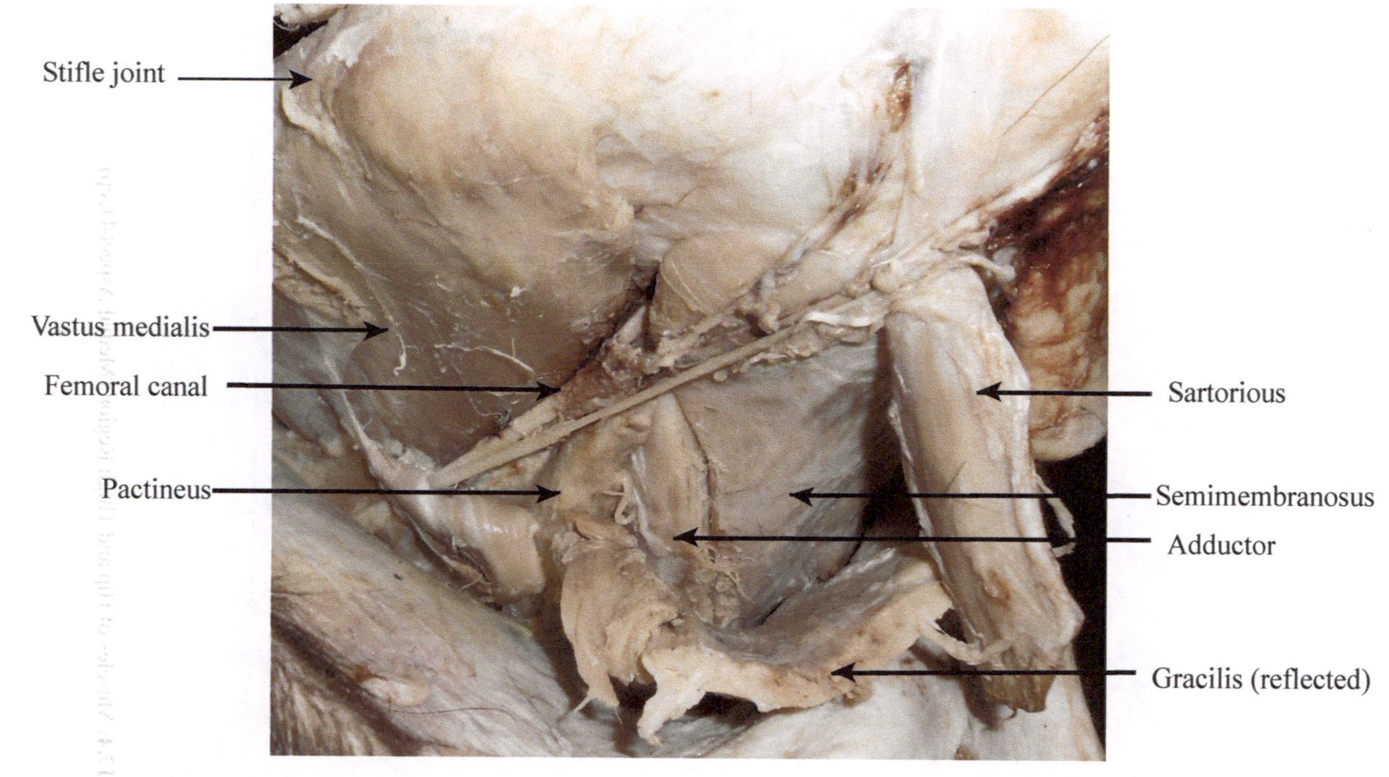

Fig. 17.3: Muscles of Hip and Thigh Region (After cutting Gracilis)

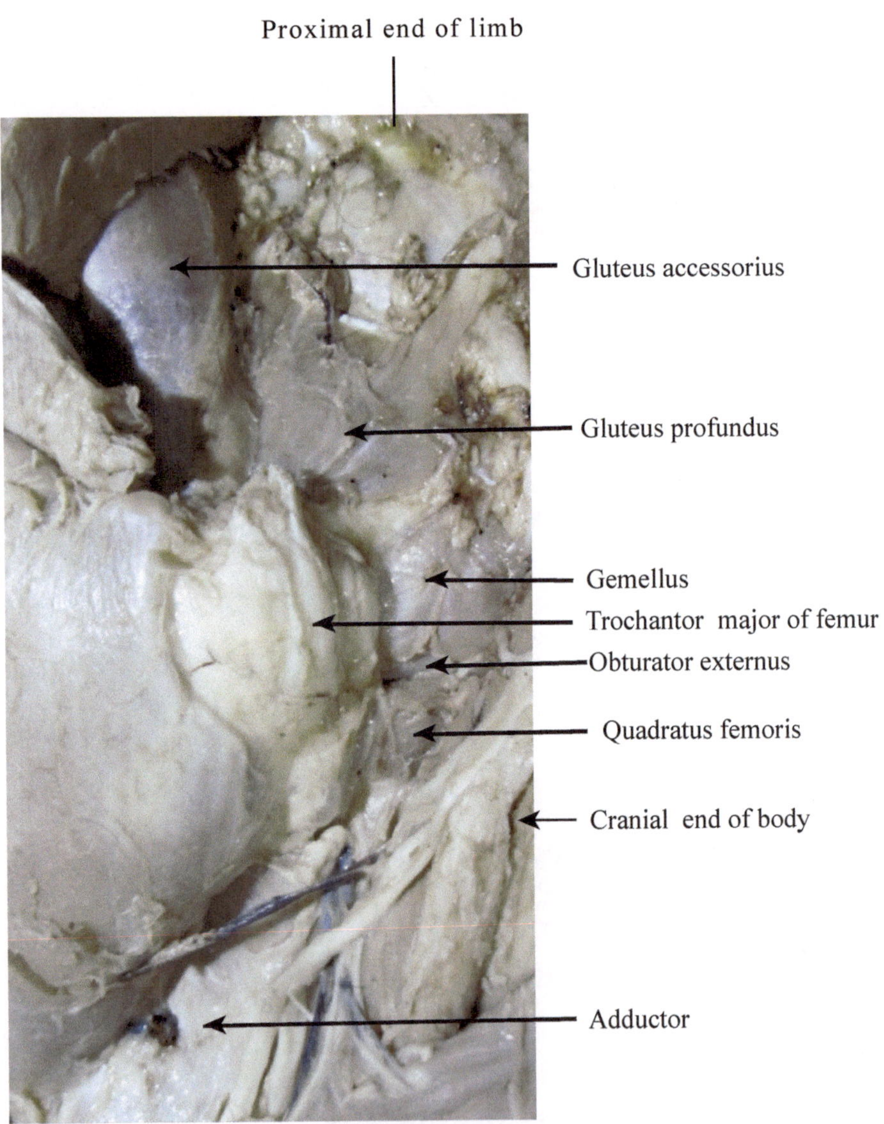

Fig.17.4: Muscles of Hip and Thigh Region (Medial Aspect-Deep)

Table 17.1: Detail of Muscles of Hip and Thigh region (Medial Aspect)

S.N.	Name of Mussle	Origin	Insestion	Action	Vessels & Nerve
1.	Semimembranosus	Ventral surface of the tuber ischii and the posterior border of the ischium	Medial epicondyle of the femur and the posterior margin of the medial condyle of the tibia.	Extent the hip and adduct the limb.	Deep femoral artery. Sciatic nerve
2.	Gracilis	Ventral border of the sub pelvic tendon and the ventral surface of the prepubic tendon close to the pubis.	Medial patellar ligament by means the tendon of the Sartorius and the medial surface of the tibia.	Adduct the limb and extend the stifle joint.	Deep femoral artery. Obturator nerve
3.	Sartorius	By the heads one from the shaft of the ilium just below the psoas tubercle and the other from the tendon of the psoas minor muscle.	Tibial tuberosity by the medial patellar ligament.	Extend the stifle and flex the hip joint.	Femoral and saphenous arteries. Saphenous nerve.
4.	Pectineus	Anterior border of the pubis and the ventral surface of the prepubic tendon.	Medial epicondyle and the medial and posterior surface of the femur above the vascular groove.	Adduct the limb and flex the hip joint	Deep femoral artery. Obturator and Saphenous nerves
5.	Adductor	Lateral surface of the subpelvic ligament and the ventral surface of the ischium.	An extensive area on the posterior surface and the medial supracondyloid crest of the femur.	To adduct the limb	Deep femoral artery Obturator nerve
6.	Obturator internus	Pelvic surface of the ischium and the symphyseal branch of the pubis.	Trochanteric fossa with the obturator extrenus.	Rotate the femur outward.	Obturator and internal pudic arteries. Sciatic nerve.
7	Obturator externus	Ventral surface of the pubis and adjacent part of the ischium and the medial margin of the obturator foramen.	Ttrochanteric fossa	Adduct the limb and rotate the femur outward	Deep femoral artery Obturator nerve
8.	Quadratus femoris	Ventral surface of the ischium near the obturator foramen	Proximal part of the posterior surface of the femur near the trochanter minor.	Extend the hip joint and adduct the limb.	Deep femoral artery Sciatic nerve
9.	Gemellus	Ischial spine, the lateral border of the ischium and the lateral surface of the tuber ischii.	Trochanteric fossa	To extend the hip joint and rotate the femur.	Posterior gluteal artery Sciatic nerve.

18

Muscles of Extensor of Digits and Flexor of Hock in Hind Limb

Site of incision: Make a mid-lateral and mid-medial longitudinal incision on hind-limb from stifle joint to 3rd digit. Joins, the above incisions transversally on cranial aspect at stifle joint and 3rd phalanx, respectively. Remove the skin on dorsolateral aspect of limb.

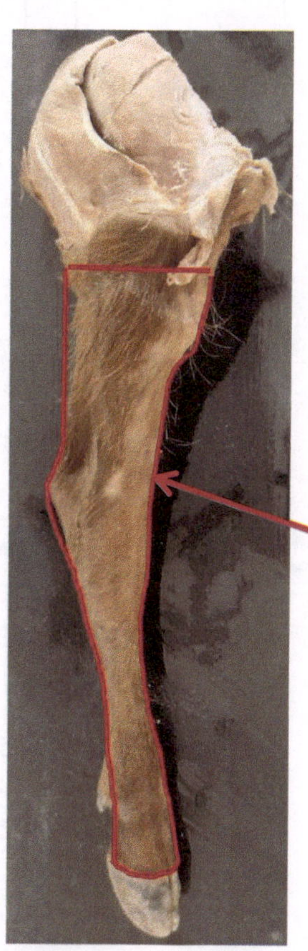

Fig. 18.1: Site of Incision (Arrow)

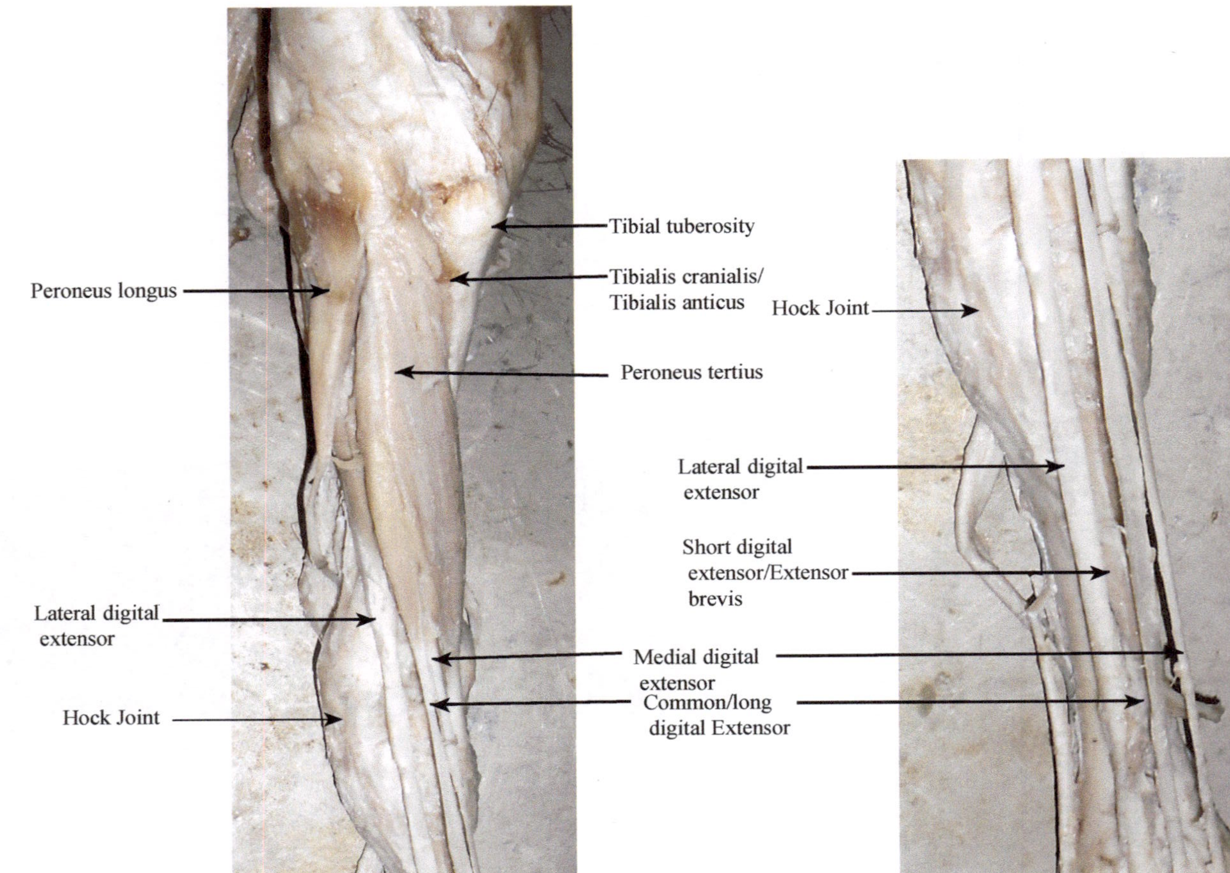

Fig. 18.2: Muscles of Extensor of Digits and Flexor of Hock in Hind Limb

Table 18.1: Detail of Muscles of Extensor of Digits and Flexor of Hock in Hind Limb

S.N	Name of muscle	Origin	Insertion	Action	Blood and Nerve supply
1.	Tibialis anterior/ cranialis	Tibial tuberosity and adjacent part of the tibial crest, the fibrous fibula and the lower margin of the sulcus muscularis.	The proximal extremity of the large metatarsal bone and the fused second and third tarsal bones	Flex the hock	Anterior tibial artery. Deep peroneal nerve.
2.	Peroneus longus	Proximal extremity (head) of the fibula and the fibrous band representing the shaft of the fibula and the lateral femoro-tibial ligament.	The first tarsal bone.	Flex the hock joint.	Anterior tibial artery. Deep peroneal nerve.
3.	Peroneus tertius	Extensor fossa of the femur with the long and medial digital extensor muscles.	Large metatarsal bone and the fused second and third tarsal bones.	Flex the hock joint. It also has a slight extension action on the stifle joint	Anterior tibial artery Deep peroneal nerve.
4.	Long digital extensor	Extensor fossa of the femur	Extensor process of the third phalanx of the third and fourth digits.	Extend the functional digits, a slight extensor action on the stifle and possibly to flex the hock.	Anterior tibial artery Deep peroneal nerve
5.	Short digital extensor (extensor brevis)	A depression on the dorsal surface of the tibial tarsal bone.	The tendon of long digital extensor in distal fourth of metatarsus.	Assist long digital extensor muscle in extending the digit	Anterior tibial and dorsal metatarsal arteries. Deep peroneal nerve.
6.	Medial digital extensor	Extensor fossa of the femur.	Dorsal surface of second and third phalanx of the third digit	Extend and abduct the third digit.	Anterior tibial artery Deep peroneal nerve
7.	Lateral digital extensor	Lateral femoro tibial ligament and the proximal extremity of the fibula.	Dorsal surface of the second and third phalanx of the fourth digit.	Extend and abduct the fourth digit	Anterior tibial artery. Superficial peroneal nerve.

19

Muscles of Flexor of Digits and Extensor of Hock in Hind Limb

Site of incision: Make a mid-lateral and mid-medial longitudinal incision on hindlimb from stiffle joint to 3rd digit. Joins the above incisions transversally on caudal aspect at stiffle joint above and 3rd phalanx below, respectively. Remove the skin on plantero-medial aspect of limb.

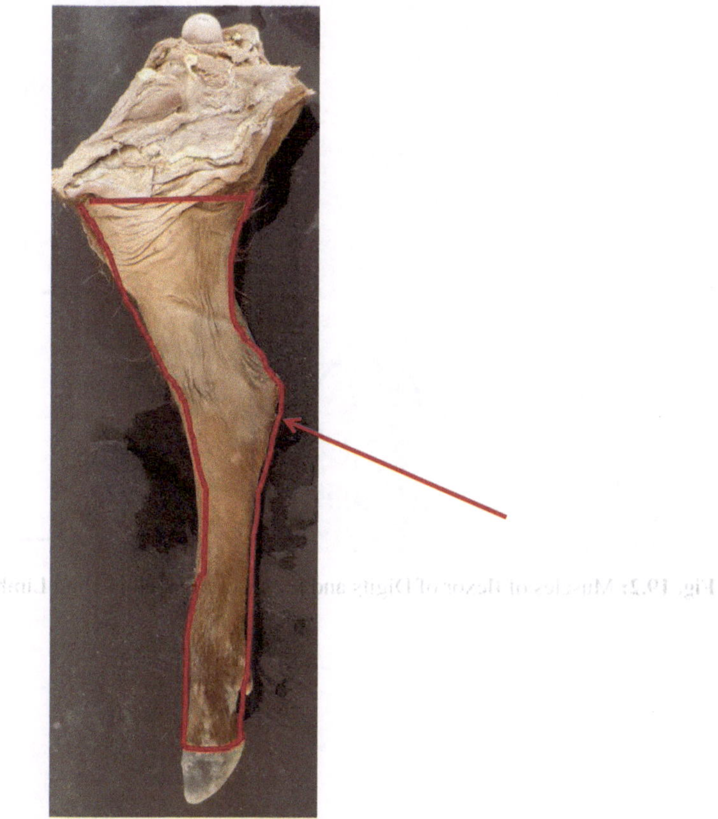

Fig. 19.1: Site of Incision (Arrow)

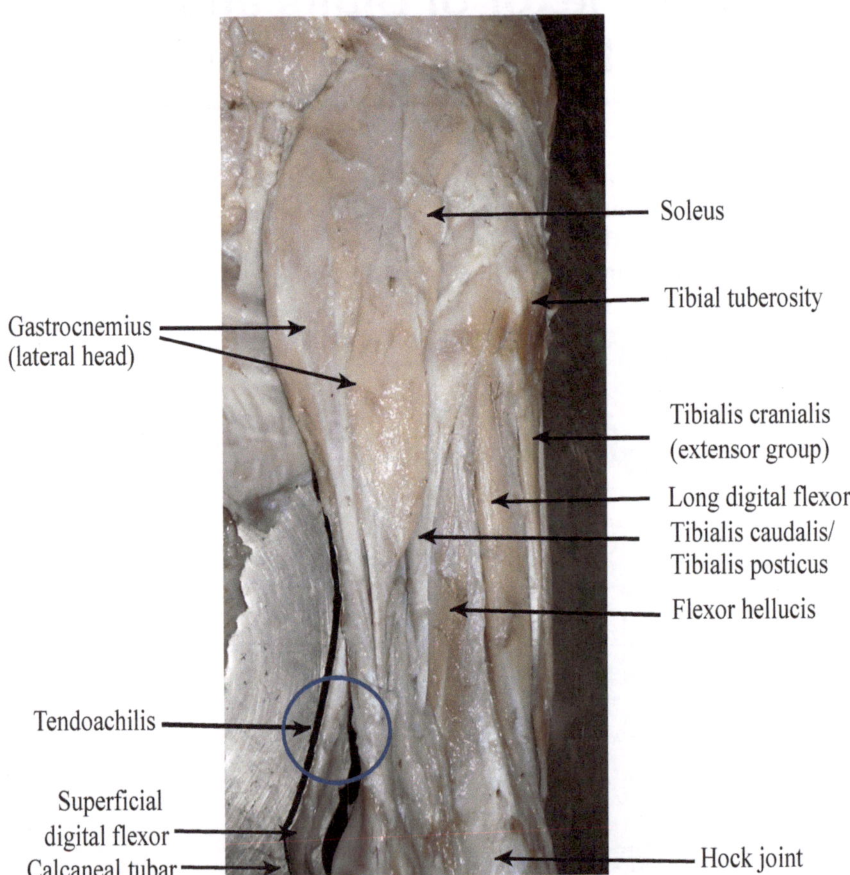

Fig. 19.2: Muscles of flexor of Digits and Extensor of Hock in Hind Limb

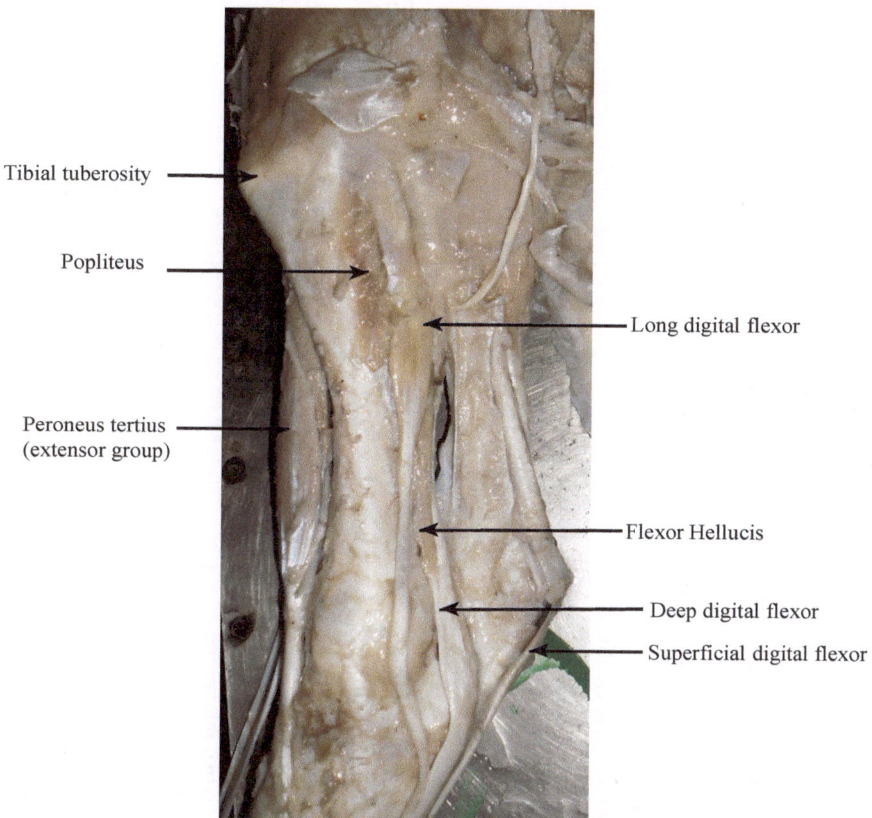

Fig. 19.3: Muscles of Flexor of Digits and Extensor of Hock in Hind Limb

Table 19.1: Muscles of Flexor of Digits and Extensor of Hock in Hind Limb

S.N	Name of muscle	Origin	Insertion	Action	Blood and Nerve supply
1.	Gastrocnemius (Medial & Lateral head)	Medial supracondyloid crest and medial epicondyle and the lateral supracondyloid crest of the femur	Anterior and proximal surface of the tuber calcis.	Extend the hock joint and flex the stifle joint. The chief action is on the hock joint.	Popliteal and posterior femoral arteries. Tibial nerve.
2	Soleus	Posterior border of the proximal extremity of the fibula and adjacent part of the lateral tibial condyle.	Tendon of the lateral head of the gastrocnemius.	To assist the gastrocnemius in extending the hock.	Popliteal artery. Tibial artery.
3.	Superficial digital flexor (3 heads)	Supracondyloid fossa of the femur.	Tuber calcis and the plantar border of the proximal extremity of the second phalanx of both functional digits.	Flex the digit, extend the hock and flex the stifle.	Popliteal artery. Tibial nerve
4.	Deep digital flexor	All three heads (1. hallucis; 2. tibialis Posticus 3. long digital flexor) have an origin on the posterior border of lateral tibial condyle. The deep head (flexor hallucis) has an origin from the proximal two-third of the plantar surface except for the area occupied by the popliteus muscle.	Thick posterior border of the plantar surface of the third phalanges of the third and fourth digits.	Flex the entire digit on the metatarsus, flex the coffin joint and, indirectly to extend the hock.	Popliteal and posterior tibial arteries. Tibial nerve.
5.	Popliteus	Popliteal fossa of the femur	Upper half of the medial borders and narrow adjacent parts of the posterior and medial surfaces of the tibia above and medial to the muscular lines.	Flex the stifle joint and possibly a slight inward protection of the leg.	Popliteal artery Tibial nerve.

20

Muscles of Tail

Site of incision: Make two incisions at mid-lateral aspect at base of the tail join them dorso-ventrally and reflect the skin caudally up the 4-5 inches.

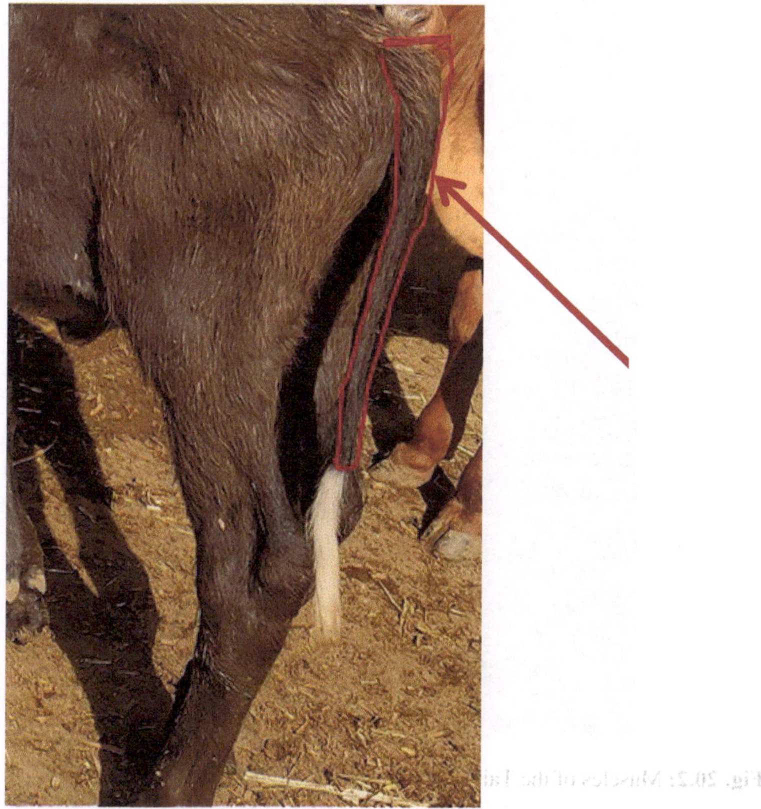

Fig. 20.1: Site of Incision (Arrow)

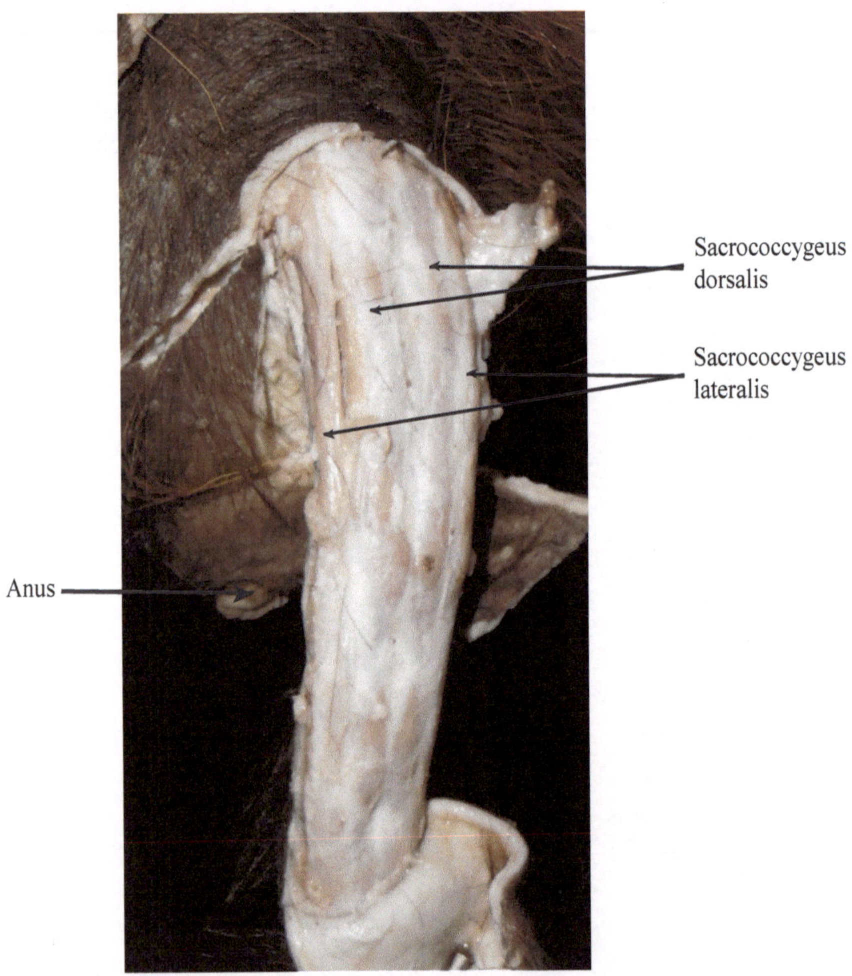

Fig. 20.2: Muscles of the Tail

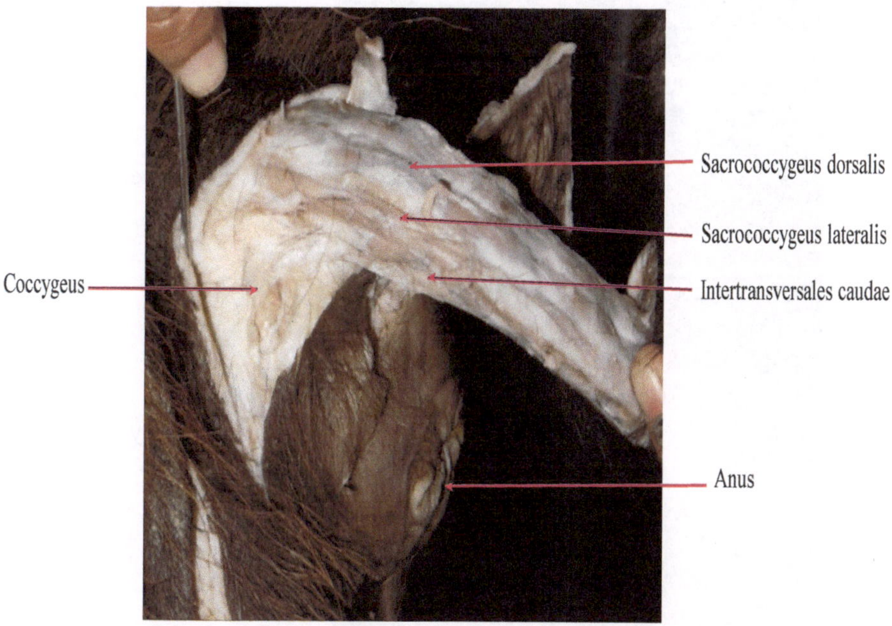

Fig. 20.3: Muscles of the Tail (dorsolateral aspect)

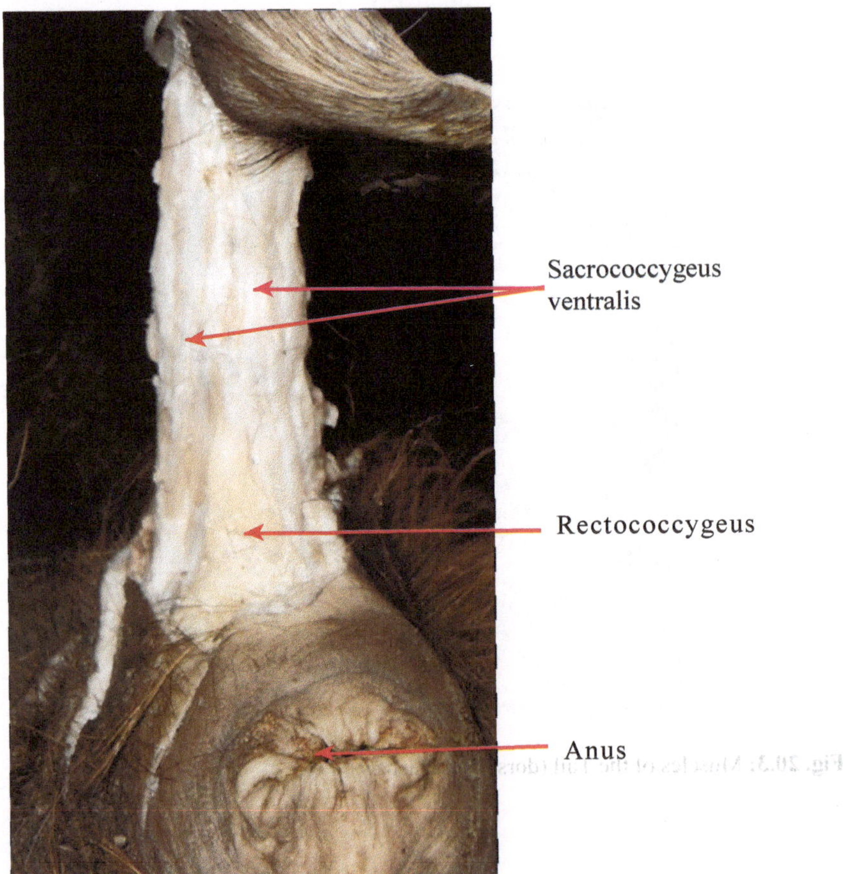

Fig. 20.4: Muscles of the Tail (Ventral aspect)

Table 20.1: Muscles of Tail

S.N	Name of muscle	Origin	Insertion	Action	Blood and Nerve supply
1.	Coccygeus	Deep surface of the sacrosciatic ligament near the ischiatic spine	Transverse processes of the second and third coccygeal vertebrae	To depress the root of the tail or incline it laterally	The middle or ventral coccygeal artery. Four or five pairs of coccygeal nerves.
2.	Sacrococcygeus dorsalis	Lateral surface of sacral spines and the lateral sacral crest and tendinous fibers in the lumbar area in common with multifidus dorsi.	Dorsal surface of caudal vertebrae	Extensors of tail	Caudal branches and dorsolateral caudal artery Caudal (spinal) nerve
3.	Sacrococcygeus lateralis	Tendons in common with longissimus dorsi	Transverse process and spine and lateral surface of caudal vertebrae	Extension and lateral flexion of tail	Caudal branches and dorsolateral caudal artery Caudal (spinal) nerve
4a.	Sacrococcygeus ventralis (lateral part)	Lateral part of ventral surface of sacrum as far craniad as 3rd pelvic sacral foramen	Transverse processes and ventral surface of all caudal vertebrae	Flexion of tail and lateral movement	Ventrolateral caudal artery Caudal (spinal) nerve
b.	Sacrococcygeus ventralis (medial part)	Ventral surface of sacrum medial to lateral part	Ventral surface of caudal vertebrae	Flexion of tail and lateral movement	Median sacral and median caudal arteries Caudal (spinal) nerve
5	Intertransversales caudae	Consist of muscular band which lie on the lateral aspect of tail,between sacrococcygeus lateralis and sacrococcygeus ventralis. They originate from lateral edges of sacrum and occupying spaces between transverse processes to which they are attached.		Fix coccygeal vertebrae and lateral flexion of the tail	Dorsolateral and ventrolateral caudal arteries Caudal (spinal) nerve
6	Rectococcygeus	It is in the form of large band, detached on either side from muscular coat of rectum, passes upward and backward to be inserted into the 4th and 5th coccygeal vertebrae.